MRCP 1
POCKET BOOK
4

Clinical Pharmacology, Immunology, Infectious Diseases and Rheumatology

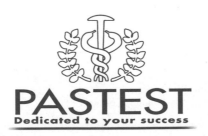

PASTEST
Dedicated to your success

© 2002 PASTEST LTD
Egerton Court, Parkgate Estate,
Knutsford, Cheshire, WA16 8DX

First edition 2002
Reprinted 2002

ISBN: 1 901198 901

A catalogue record for this book is available from the British Library.

The information contained within this book was obtained by the author from reliable sources. However, while every effort has been made to ensure its accuracy, no responsibilty for loss, damage or injury occasioned to any person acting or refraining from action as a result of information contained herein can be accepted by the publishers or author.

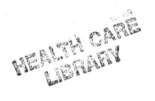

Typeset by Breeze Limited, Manchester
Printed by MPG Books Ltd., Bodmin, Cornwall

CONTENTS

14 858

INTRODUCTION

PasTest's MRCP Part 1 Pocket Books are designed to help the busy examination candidate to make the most of every opportunity to revise. With this little book in your pocket, it is the work of a moment to open it, choose a question, decide upon your answers and then check the answer. Revising 'on the run' in this manner is both reassuring (if your answer is correct) and stimulating (if you find any gaps in your knowledge).

For quite some time the Royal College of Physicians has been conducting an extensive review of the MRCP Part 1 examination and has recently announced changes to be introduced in May 2002. From an educational point of view both these changes are to be welcomed.

Negative marking (penalty scoring) will be discontinued
From the candidates' point of view, this is an important change because incorrect answers will no longer be penalised by the deduction of marks – they will simply not gain any marks. (From the Examiners' point of view it should improve the reliability of the examination by removing an uncontrollable variable – individual candidates' willingness to venture an answer when they are less than 100% confident.)

A second paper will be introduced in addition to the current 2½ hour, 60 question multiple true/false examination. This will also last for 2½ hours, but consist of 100 questions using a new type of Multiple Choice Question (MCQ) – the one-best answer/'Best of Five' format.
This means that the examination from May 2002 onwards will last all day. Candidates will also need to become familiar with one-best MCQs and the strategies for answering them. However, one-best is a much better design than multiple true/false. They are typically more valid and reliable, so their introduction should be to the advantage of good candidates.

One-best answer/'Best of Five' MCQs
An important characteristic of one-best answer MCQs is that they can be designed to test application of knowledge and clinical problem-solving rather than just the recall of facts. This should change (for the better) the ways in which candidates prepare for MRCP Part 1.

Each one-best MCQ has a question stem, which usually contains clinical information, followed by five branches. All five branches are typically homologous (e.g. all diagnoses, all laboratory investigations, all antibiotics etc) and should be set out in a logical order (e.g. alphabetical). Candidates are asked to select the ONE branch that is the best answer to the question. A response is not required to the other four branches. The answer sheet is, therefore, slightly different to that used for true/false MCQs.

A good strategy that can be used with many well-written one-best MCQs is to try to reach the correct answer without first scrutinising the five options. If you can then find the answer you have reached in the option list, then you are probably correct.

One-best answer MCQs are quicker to answer than multiple true/false MCQs because only one response is needed for each question. Even though the question stem for one-best answer MCQs is usually longer than for true/false questions, and therefore takes a little longer to read carefully, it is reasonable to set more one-best than true/false MCQs for the same exam duration – in this instance 60 true/false and 100 one-best are used in exams of 2 hours.

Application of Knowledge and Clinical Problem-Solving
Unlike true/false MCQs, which test mainly the recall of knowledge, one-best answer questions test application and problem-solving. This makes them more effective test items and is one of the reasons why testing time can be reduced. In order to answer these questions correctly, it is necessary to apply basic knowledge – not just be able to remember it. Furthermore, candidates who cannot reach the correct answer by applying their knowledge are much less likely to be able to choose the right answer by guessing than they were with true/false MCQs. This gives a big advantage to the best candidates, who have good knowledge and can apply it in clinical situations.

Multiple Choice Questions
Each question consists of an initial statement followed by five possible completions, ABCDE. There is no restriction on the number of true or false items in a question. It is possible for all items in a question to be true or for all to be false. The most important points of technique are:
1. Read the question carefully and be sure you understand it.
2. Mark your response clearly, correctly and accurately.
3. The best possible way to obtain a good mark is to have as wide a knowledge as possible of the topics being tested in the examination.

To get the best value from the MCQ sections you should commit yourself to an answer for each item before you check the correct answer. It is only by being sure of your own responses that you can ascertain which questions you would find difficult in the examination.

Books like the ones in this series, which consist of 'Best of Five' and MCQs in subject categories, can help you to focus on specific topics and to isolate your weaknesses. You should plan a revision timetable to help you spread your time evenly over the range of subjects likely to appear in the examination. PasTest's Essential Revision Notes for MRCP by P Kalra will provide you with essential notes on all aspects of the syllabus.

CLINICAL PHARMACOLOGY

'Best of Five' and MCQs

Prof M Pirmohamed PhD, FRCP, FRCP (Edin)
Professor of Clinical Pharmacology
and Hon Consultant Physician
Department of Pharmacology and Therapeutics
The University of Liverpool
Liverpool

CLINICAL PHARMACOLOGY: 'BEST OF FIVE' QUESTIONS

For each of the questions select the ONE most appropriate answer from the options provided.

1.1   Which one of the following actions is mediated by the α-adrenoceptor?

- ❏   A   Bronchiolar constriction
- ❏   B   Decrease in gut motility
- ❏   C   Dilatation of the splanchnic circulation
- ❏   D   Penile erection
- ❏   E   Relaxation of pregnant uterus

1.2   Zanamivir in the treatment of influenza is characterised by all of the following EXCEPT?

- ❏   A   A bioavailability of less than 20%
- ❏   B   A decrease in bronchial air flow
- ❏   C   Increased release of virus from cells
- ❏   D   Reduced penetration of the virus into the respiratory mucosa
- ❏   E   Reduced severity of the illness

1.3   Cephalosporins

- ❏   A   Can be used in the treatment of *Clostridium difficile* diarrhoea
- ❏   B   Can cause neutropenia and thrombocytopenia
- ❏   C   Do not have a β-lactam ring in their structure
- ❏   D   Have a 90% chance of causing allergy if the patient has had a previous reaction to penicillin
- ❏   E   In general have half-lives greater than 10 hours

1.4   Which one of the following causes of hypercalcaemia is most likely to respond to treatment with corticosteroids?

- ❏   A   Milk-alkali syndrome
- ❏   B   Paget's disease
- ❏   C   Primary hyperparathyroidism
- ❏   D   Sarcoidosis
- ❏   E   Small cell lung cancer

1.5   In relation to morphine, which one of the following statements is true?

- ❏ A   Approximately 8% of the population cannot convert codeine to morphine
- ❏ B   Morphine is more water-soluble than diamorphine
- ❏ C   Normal release morphine has an onset of action within 5 minutes
- ❏ D   Peak drug levels after once daily preparations of morphine are reached after 12 hours
- ❏ E   Pupillary constriction is an effect that is subject to tolerance

1.6   Regarding β-adrenoceptor antagonists

- ❏ A   Atenolol is a cardio-specific drug
- ❏ B   Celiprolol increases total peripheral resistance
- ❏ C   Drugs with intrinsic sympathomimetic activity are less likely to cause bradycardia
- ❏ D   Esmolol is a long-acting drug used to treat patients with atrial arrhythmias
- ❏ E   Propranolol causes prolongation of the Q-T interval

1.7   Which one of the following is a known effect of the anticonvulsant phenytoin?

- ❏ A   Can cause selective IgA deficiency
- ❏ B   Causes arrhythmias in 10% of patients
- ❏ C   Displays first-order kinetics
- ❏ D   Efficacy in myoclonic epilepsy
- ❏ E   Osteoporosis is a known adverse effect

1.8   The following are well known drug-drug interactions; which one of these can be considered to be a beneficial interaction and has been used therapeutically?

- ❏ A   Cimetidine and dapsone
- ❏ B   Cimetidine and phenytoin
- ❏ C   Cisapride and erythromycin
- ❏ D   Rifampicin and cyclosporin A
- ❏ E   Ritonavir and fluoxetine

1.9 **Severe poisoning with iron is characterised by which one of the following?**

- ❏ A Blood glucose > 8.3 mmol/l
- ❏ B Hypertension
- ❏ C Normal plain abdominal X-ray
- ❏ D Pulmonary haemorrhage
- ❏ E Total white cell count of < 4 x 10^9/l

1.10 **Which one of the following statements relating to the use of acetylcholinesterase inhibitors in the treatment of Alzheimer's disease is true?**

- ❏ B Donepezil binds to the esteratic site of the enzyme
- ❏ E Donepezil has a half-life of 7 hours
- ❏ A Metrifonate binds reversibly to the active site of the enzyme
- ❏ C Rivastigmine binds to both the anionic and esteratic sites of the enzyme
- ❏ D The metabolite of metrifonate does not possess any pharmacological activity

1.11 **Below is a list of drugs with their putative adverse reactions. Which one of the pairings is not correct?**

- ❏ A Cerivastatin – rhabdomyolysis
- ❏ B Indinavir – renal stones
- ❏ C Pergolide – pulmonary fibrosis
- ❏ D Tolcapone – neuroleptic malignant syndrome
- ❏ E Vigabatrin – anterior uveitis

1.12 **Which one of the following statements about leflunomide is incorrect?**

- ❏ A It can be classed as a disease-modifying anti-rheumatic drug
- ❏ B It has active metabolites
- ❏ C It has comparable efficacy to sulfasalazine and methotrexate
- ❏ D It inhibits dihydroorotate dehydrogenase
- ❏ E It inhibits purine synthesis

1.13   During warfarin therapy which one of the following statements is correct?

❑   A   Dosage is adjusted by monitoring drug levels

❑   B   Dose requirements are genetically determined

❑   C   Osteoporosis may develop

❑   D   Overdose can be reversed by protamine sulphate

❑   E   Therapeutic effect is usually achieved within 24 hours

1.14   When inducing local anaesthesia by infiltration which one of the following is correct?

❑   A   Accidental injection of lignocaine into the systemic circulation may increase myocardial and neuronal excitability

❑   B   Bupivacaine produces a shorter lasting anaesthesia than lignocaine

❑   C   The anaesthetic agents used are strongly acidic

❑   D   The duration of anaesthesia may be prolonged by the addition of salbutamol

❑   E   The duration of anaesthesia with lignocaine depends on diffusion and not on drug metabolism

1.15   Which one of the following statements regarding combined hormonal oral contraceptives is incorrect?

❑   A   Oestrogen preparations promote blood clotting

❑   B   Oestrogens inhibit follicle stimulating hormone release

❑   C   Progestogens inhibit luteinising hormone release

❑   D   The incidence of benign breast disease may be increased

❑   E   The risk of stroke is increased to a small extent

1.16   In relation to the use of interferon beta in the treatment of multiple sclerosis, which one of the following is incorrect?

❑   A   Does not have a beneficial effect if administered at the time of the first ever demyelinating event

❑   B   Reduces brain atrophy

❑   C   Reduces relapses in patients with chronic multiple sclerosis

❑   D   Reduces the development of brain lesions on MRI

❑   E   Slows progression of physical disability

1.17 **Which one of the following antidepressants is least likely to cause anticholinergic side effects?**

- ❏ A   Amitriptyline
- ❏ B   Clomipramine
- ❏ C   Dothiepin
- ❏ D   Lofepramine
- ❏ E   Trazodone

1.18 **Concerning Sumatriptan**

- ❏ A   Bioavailability after oral and subcutaneous administration is equivalent
- ❏ B   It can be used safely in patients with known coronary artery disease
- ❏ C   It can be used together with ergotamine in migraine
- ❏ D   It inhibits the release of calcitonin gene-related peptide
- ❏ E   It prevents the aura associated with migraine

1.19 **Concerning Bupropion**

- ❏ A   It can cause Stevens-Johnson syndrome
- ❏ B   It is a selective inhibitor of the neuronal uptake of noradrenaline
- ❏ C   It is an enzyme inhibitor
- ❏ D   It is effective in smoking cessation
- ❏ E   It should not be used in patients with a history of seizures

1.20 **Which one of the following CNS active drugs should be avoided in breast-feeding mothers?**

- ❏ A   Codeine
- ❏ B   Hyoscine
- ❏ C   Neostigmine
- ❏ D   Oxcarbazepine
- ❏ E   Propranolol

1.21   Which one of the following drugs is not used to treat minimal change glomerulonephritis?

❑   A   Chlorambucil

❑   B   Cyclophosphamide

❑   C   Cyclosporin

❑   D   Prednisolone

❑   E   Vincristine

1.22   In relation to analgesic nephropathy, which one of the following statements is correct?

❑   A   Analgesic nephropathy was previously the commonest cause of renal failure in Australia

❑   B   Onset of analgesic nephropathy is common after a week of heavy analgesic use

❑   C   Phenacetin has not been implicated in the aetiology of analgesic nephropathy

❑   D   Renal transplantation is contraindicated in cases of analgesic nephropathy

❑   E   The renal lesion in analgesic nephropathy is unique

1.23   Which one of the following statements is not correct in relation to the nephrotoxicity of drugs?

❑   A   Aminoglycosides cause proximal tubular necrosis

❑   B   Amphotericin B reduces renal blood flow

❑   C   Analgesic nephropathy is characterized pathologically by glomerulonephritis

❑   D   Gold is associated with glomerulonephritis

❑   E   Lithium carbonate causes nephrogenic diabetes insipidus

1.24   With respect to therapeutic drug monitoring for a patient with renal failure, which one of the following statements is correct?

❏   A   Concomitant administration of diuretics makes aminoglycoside toxicity more likely

❏   B   Steady state levels of theophylline can be measured after 2 half-lives of the drug

❏   C   The only way to avoid toxicity is to reduce the dose of a potentially toxic drug

❏   D   Therapeutic concentrations of vancomycin are unlikely to be maintained beyond 24 hours after dosage

❏   E   When giving gentamicin, a trough level is sufficient to determine dosage adjustment

1.25   Which one of the following drugs does NOT cause constipation?

❏   A   Cholestyramine

❏   B   Disopyramide

❏   C   Nifedipine

❏   D   Tricyclic antidepressants (TCA)

❏   E   Verapamil

1.26   A 67-year-old gentleman with a history of alcohol excess is admitted for the third time with a large haematemesis due to proven oesophageal varices. Which one of the following therapies has been shown to reduce mortality in the acute situation?

❏   A   Antibiotics

❏   B   Glypressin

❏   C   Intravenous ranitidine

❏   D   Octreotide

❏   E   Propranolol

1.27 **Which one of the following drugs can safely be used in liver failure without dose adjustment?**

- ❑ A Digoxin
- ❑ B Erythromycin
- ❑ C Metformin
- ❑ D Morphine
- ❑ E Propranolol

1.28 **When considering paracetamol overdose, which one of the following is LEAST likely to increase the risk of liver damage occurring?**

- ❑ A Acute alcohol intake
- ❑ B Anorexia nervosa
- ❑ C Concomitant therapy with isoniazid
- ❑ D Concomitant therapy with phenytoin
- ❑ E HIV positive diagnosis

1.29 **Methotrexate acts by**

- ❑ A Binding to DNA
- ❑ B Increasing the metabolism of folic acid derivatives
- ❑ C Inhibition of dihydrofolate oxidase
- ❑ D Inhibiting DNA polymerase
- ❑ E Reducing nucleotide biosynthesis

1.30 **Lung fibrosis can be caused by**

- ❑ A 5-Fluorouracil
- ❑ B Busulphan
- ❑ C Cyclophosphamide
- ❑ D Cytarabine
- ❑ E Vincristine

1.31   **During the cell cycle, 5-fluorouracil exerts its actions predominantly during**
- ❑ A   Cell differentiation
- ❑ B   The G0 phase
- ❑ C   The G1 and S phases
- ❑ D   The G2 and M phases
- ❑ E   The S and G2 phases

1.32   **Hydroxyurea is commonly used in the treatment of which one of the following?**
- ❑ A   Acute lymphocytic leukaemia
- ❑ B   Breast carcinoma
- ❑ C   Carcinoma of the cervix
- ❑ D   Chronic myeloid leukaemia
- ❑ E   Non-Hodgkins lymphoma

1.33   **In patients with suspected acute intermittent porphyria, which one of the following drugs should be avoided?**
- ❑ A   Amoxycillin
- ❑ B   Dapsone
- ❑ C   Gentamicin
- ❑ D   Griseofulvin
- ❑ E   Tetracycline

1.34   **Which one of the following may help reduce insulin resistance?**
- ❑ A   Acarbose
- ❑ B   Atenolol
- ❑ C   High dose Bendrofluazide
- ❑ D   Metformin
- ❑ E   Prednisolone

1.35 **Which one of the following is true of the Selective Estrogen Receptor Modulator (SERM), raloxifene?**

  ❑ A   Associated with an increased risk of breast carcinoma

  ❑ B   Is extensively renally excreted

  ❑ C   Reduces the risk of non-vertebral body fractures

  ❑ D   Reduces the risk of vertebral fractures by 30%

  ❑ E   Results in vaginal bleeding

1.36 **In a hypertensive patient with diabetic nephropathy which one of the following should be the drug of first choice?**

  ❑ A   Atenolol

  ❑ B   Bendrofluazide

  ❑ C   Captopril

  ❑ D   Diltiazem

  ❑ E   Doxazosin

CLINICAL PHARMACOLOGY: MULTIPLE CHOICE QUESTIONS

Mark your answers with a tick (True) or a cross (False) in the box provided.

1.37 **Inhibition of protein synthesis is the mode of action of the following antibiotics:**

☐ A   chloramphenicol

☐ B   penicillin

☐ C   ciprofloxacin

☐ D   gentamicin

☐ E   teicoplanin

1.38 **In the treatment of insulin-dependent diabetes mellitus (IDDM)**

☐ A   effective control of blood sugar has been shown to decrease long-term complications

☐ B   insulin lispro has a slower onset of action than soluble insulin

☐ C   insulin lispro lowers glycosylated haemoglobin

☐ D   porcine insulin is more immunogenic than human insulin

☐ E   patients should reduce their insulin dosage if they develop an intercurrent infection

1.39 **Tamoxifen**

☐ A   is more effective in postmenopausal women with breast cancer than in premenopausal women

☐ B   is known to reduce the risk of endometrial cancer

☐ C   can cause retinopathy

☐ D   can result in hypercalcaemia

☐ E   is a pure antagonist at oestrogen receptors

1.40   Regarding the use of protease inhibitors in HIV disease

☐ A   they inhibit the viral serine protease

☐ B   in combination with nucleoside analogues, they retard disease progression and decrease mortality

☐ C   non-compliance may lead to the development of resistance

☐ D   they interact with rifabutin and increase the risk of uveitis

☐ E   they are associated with the development of lipodystrophy

1.41   The following drugs have proven teratogenic effects in humans:

☐ A   diazepam

☐ B   misoprostol

☐ C   warfarin

☐ D   oral contraceptives

☐ E   aspirin

1.42   Regarding hormone replacement therapy (HRT)

☐ A   unopposed oestrogens can be used in patients who have had a hysterectomy

☐ B   it is associated with an increased risk of venous thromboembolism

☐ C   non-steroidal drugs such as raloxifene can also be used

☐ D   use may be associated with protection against Alzheimer's disease

☐ E   the benefits on bone are the same irrespective of when the drugs are started after the menopause

1.43   Regarding the management of drug overdose

☐ A   gastric lavage should be used up to six hours after the overdose

☐ B   ipecacuanha syrup should be used in children

☐ C   activated charcoal reduces the entero-hepatic circulation of drugs

☐ D   haemodialysis is useful for eliminating drugs with a high volume of distribution

☐ E   alkalinisation of urine can be used to increase the elimination of acidic drugs

1.44 Grapefruit juice interacts with the following drugs:

- ❏ A felodipine
- ❏ B cisapride
- ❏ C atenolol
- ❏ D saquinavir
- ❏ E sodium valproate

1.45 Regarding the process of drug metabolism the following statements are correct:

- ❏ A the primary role of drug metabolism is to convert hydrophilic compounds into lipophilic compounds
- ❏ B drugs can be metabolised in the gut wall
- ❏ C metabolism can result in the formation of toxic metabolites with some compounds
- ❏ D cytochrome P450 enzymes are largely responsible for the phase II metabolic pathways
- ❏ E genetically determined deficiencies of some of the drug metabolising enzymes have been described

1.46 Atypical neuroleptics in comparison with typical neuroleptics are generally

- ❏ A less likely to cause Parkinsonism
- ❏ B more likely to cause neuroleptic malignant syndrome
- ❏ C less likely to affect the negative symptoms of schizophrenia
- ❏ D less likely to affect the positive symptoms of schizophrenia
- ❏ E less likely to cause weight gain

1.47 The following anti-epileptic drugs are correctly paired with their main mode of action:

- ❏ A lamotrigine: glutamate antagonism
- ❏ B diazepam: inhibition of GABA re-uptake
- ❏ C ethosuximide: inhibition of calcium conductance
- ❏ D carbamazepine: inhibition of sodium conductance
- ❏ E tiagabine: inhibition of GABA transaminase

1.48   Lithium carbonate

- ❑   A   affects mood in normal subjects
- ❑   B   can cause nephrogenic diabetes insipidus
- ❑   C   interacts with bendrofluazide
- ❑   D   can be used in breast-feeding mothers
- ❑   E   should be avoided in patients with moderate to severe renal impairment

1.49   An acute attack of gout may be precipitated by

- ❑   A   allopurinol
- ❑   B   probenecid
- ❑   C   atenolol
- ❑   D   adenosine
- ❑   E   cyclosporin

1.50   In the use of antibiotics

- ❑   A   clindamycin is useful in the treatment of osteomyelitis because it penetrates bone well
- ❑   B   clindamycin can be used for the treatment of pseudomembranous colitis
- ❑   C   teicoplanin is effective against methicillin-resistant *Staphylococcus aureus*
- ❑   D   co-amoxiclav can cause cholestatic hepatitis
- ❑   E   clarithromycin is active against atypical mycobacteria

1.51   Regarding generic medicines

- ❑   A   demonstration of bioequivalence with the brand leader is usually required before the drug is allowed to be marketed
- ❑   B   bioequivalence with modified release preparations is readily demonstrable
- ❑   C   bioequivalence studies are usually multiple dose studies
- ❑   D   bioequivalence studies are performed in patients with the relevant diseases
- ❑   E   different brands of lithium vary widely in bioavailability and must be prescribed by brand name

1.52   The following statements are correct:

- ❏ A   a first-pass effect means that a drug only works the first time it is taken
- ❏ B   zero order kinetics mean that the rate of elimination of the drug is dependent on the plasma concentration
- ❏ C   bioavailability refers to the percentage of drug reaching the systemic circulation
- ❏ D   the terminal half-life of a drug is the time taken to excrete all of a given dose
- ❏ E   glucuronidation usually increases the lipid insolubility of a drug

1.53   Digoxin toxicity may be

- ❏ A   potentiated by hypokalaemia
- ❏ B   potentiated by hyponatraemia
- ❏ C   diagnosed by S-T elevation on the ECG
- ❏ D   treated with phenytoin
- ❏ E   treated with an infusion of calcium chloride

1.54   Riluzole

- ❏ A   acts as a glutamate agonist
- ❏ B   can only be used in amyotrophic lateral sclerosis
- ❏ C   improves functional capacity in patients with amyotrophic lateral sclerosis
- ❏ D   causes an increase in liver enzymes in more than 1 in 100 patients
- ❏ E   has been shown to improve quality of life in patients with amyotrophic lateral sclerosis

1.55   The following drugs can cause anaemia:

- ❏ A   metformin
- ❏ B   meloxicam
- ❏ C   alendronate
- ❏ D   atenolol
- ❏ E   chloramphenicol

1.56   Receptors

- ☐ A   are present on plasma membrane, in cytosol and in the nucleus
- ☐ B   initiate the pharmacological actions of all drugs
- ☐ C   actions remain constant in the continued presence of an agonist
- ☐ D   interacting with G proteins usually stimulate guanylate cyclase activity
- ☐ E   responding to insulin are linked to transmembrane protein tyrosine kinases

1.57   Regarding infection of the stomach by *Helicobacter pylori*

- ☐ A   patients with peptic ulcer have been shown to benefit from eradication therapy
- ☐ B   patients with non-specific dyspepsia have been shown to benefit from eradication therapy
- ☐ C   long-term therapy with omeprazole without antibiotics can alter the distribution of infection within the stomach
- ☐ D   the different eradication therapies are generally associated with an eradication rate of 70%
- ☐ E   it is associated with an increased risk of cancer of the gastric corpus and antrum

1.58   Regarding the use of α-interferon in patients with chronic hepatitis C virus infection

- ☐ A   a sustained response rate is seen in 50% of patients
- ☐ B   fever and myalgia are common adverse effects
- ☐ C   it can sometimes lead to bone marrow suppression
- ☐ D   response is better in patients who are currently abusing alcohol
- ☐ E   the concomitant use of paracetamol is contraindicated

1.59   Angiotensin-II receptor antagonists and angiotensin converting enzyme inhibitors share the following properties:

- ☐ A   cough as an adverse effect
- ☐ B   utility in the treatment of heart failure and hypertension
- ☐ C   blockade of the degradation of bradykinin
- ☐ D   contraindicated in patients with bilateral renal artery stenosis
- ☐ E   teratogenicity

1.60   With regard to meningococcal meningitis

- ❏ A   treatment should be withheld until cultures are taken in patients with suspected disease
- ❏ B   dexamethasone should be routinely administered in patients with septicaemia
- ❏ C   chemoprophylaxis is indicated for household and intimate contacts
- ❏ D   chemoprophylaxis is indicated for all health-care workers coming into contact with the patient
- ❏ E   treatment with ceftriaxone is superior to treatment with cefuroxime

1.61   Expected findings in salicylate poisoning in adults include

- ❏ A   tinnitus
- ❏ B   hypoglycaemia
- ❏ C   hyperventilation
- ❏ D   peptic ulceration
- ❏ E   hypoprothrombinaemia

1.62   Regarding the neuroleptic malignant syndrome

- ❏ A   it is a dose-related adverse effect of phenothiazines
- ❏ B   affected patients are fully conscious
- ❏ C   calcium channel blockers have been shown to reduce mortality
- ❏ D   it is characterised by elevated creatine phosphokinase levels
- ❏ E   it has an insidious onset

1.63   Regarding anti-arrhythmic drugs

- ❏ A   adenosine is beneficial in the treatment of atrial fibrillation
- ❏ B   digoxin toxicity can result in atrial fibrillation
- ❏ C   sotalol has both class II and class III effects
- ❏ D   propafenone has beta adrenoceptor blocking activity
- ❏ E   magnesium may be of use in patients with torsades des pointes

1.64   The following drug combinations should be avoided if possible:

❑   A   rifabutin and clarithromycin

❑   B   zidovudine and acyclovir

❑   C   isosorbide mononitrate and sildenafil

❑   D   aspirin and streptokinase

❑   E   naproxen and penicillamine

1.65   The following statements regarding adverse drug reaction (ADR) reporting in the UK are correct:

❑   A   ADR reporting is compulsory

❑   B   all serious ADRs should be reported

❑   C   a black triangle (▼) sign by a drug in the *British National Formulary* indicates that only allergic reactions need be reported

❑   D   only doctors, dentists and coroners are allowed to report on yellow cards

❑   E   yellow card reports allow a causal relationship to be established between a drug and an ADR

1.66   In relation to the apparent volume of distribution (Vd) of a drug in a 70 kg man

❑   A   Vd does not exceed the volume of total body water

❑   B   Vd would be expected to be 5 litres if the drug remained in the blood

❑   C   overdose of a drug with a low Vd can be treated by haemodialysis

❑   D   Vd is low if the drug is avidly bound in the tissues

❑   E   Vd can be calculated from a knowledge of the dose and concentration in plasma if the drug has linear kinetics

1.67   Concerning pyridoxine (vitamin B_6)

❑   A   vitamin B_6 status can be assessed by the tryptophan loading test

❑   B   prolonged use of penicillamine can lead to vitamin B_6 deficiency

❑   C   its use is contraindicated in pregnant women

❑   D   it should not be given to patients with Parkinson's disease being treated with L-dopa and carbidopa

❑   E   it is extensively metabolised within the liver

1.68   Regarding the use of anti-thyroid drugs, the following statements are correct:

❏   A   propylthiouracil inhibits the peripheral conversion of T_4 to T_3

❏   B   beta-blockers reduce the basal metabolic rate

❏   C   carbimazole produces an improvement in 2 days

❏   D   iodide can cause a goitre in euthyroid patients

❏   E   radioactive iodine (^{131}I) predominantly emits γ rays

1.69   Regarding poisoning with methanol

❏   A   the major route of elimination of methanol is by oxidation in the liver

❏   B   optic atrophy occurs within a few days

❏   C   monitoring of blood levels is important in the management of poisoning

❏   D   metabolic acidosis with a normal anion gap is the usual finding

❏   E   ethanol prevents methanol toxicity by inhibiting its oxidation within the liver

1.70   Flushing is commonly observed when alcohol is administered with the following drugs:

❏   A   procarbazine

❏   B   chlorpropamide

❏   C   disulfiram

❏   D   metronidazole

❏   E   naltrexone

1.71   Resistance to penicillins is present in 20% or more of isolates of the following bacterial species:

❏   A   *Escherichia coli*

❏   B   *Neisseria meningitidis*

❏   C   beta-haemolytic streptococci

❏   D   *Enterobacter*

❏   E   *Haemophilus influenzae*

1.72   Low molecular weight heparins in comparison to unfractionated heparin are

- ❏ A   weaker inhibitors of thrombin
- ❏ B   more likely to have reduced clearance in patients with renal failure
- ❏ C   less likely to cause bleeding
- ❏ D   more likely to cause thrombocytopenia
- ❏ E   less likely to cause osteoporosis during long-term administration

1.73   Regarding the use of aromatase inhibitors in breast cancer

- ❏ A   anastrazole is a more potent and selective inhibitor when compared to aminoglutethimide
- ❏ B   corticosteroid replacement is necessary in patients on aminoglutethimide
- ❏ C   anastrazole affects adrenal function
- ❏ D   they are efficacious in pre- and post-menopausal women
- ❏ E   inhibition of aromatase occurs predominantly within the ovaries rather than in the extra-glandular sites

1.74   The following statements regarding obesity and its treatment are correct:

- ❏ A   appetite suppressant medications can lead to primary pulmonary hypertension
- ❏ B   heart valve regurgitation has been shown to be associated with treatment with fenfluramine and phentermine
- ❏ C   mitral stenosis occurs in association with the use of fenfluramine and phentermine
- ❏ D   selective serotonin re-uptake inhibitors (SSRIs) cause heart valve abnormalities
- ❏ E   obesity *per se* is associated with a high prevalence of heart valve regurgitation

1.75   Drugs that may induce priapism in men include

- ❏ A   trazodone
- ❏ B   imipramine
- ❏ C   prazosin
- ❏ D   propranolol
- ❏ E   chlorpromazine

1.76   Sodium valproate

❏   A   should not be used in patients with myoclonic epilepsy

❏   B   increases the risk of lamotrigine-induced skin rashes

❏   C   can cause severe liver toxicity which is more common in children than
            in adults

❏   D   causes weight loss

❏   E   causes pancreatitis

IMMUNOLOGY

'Best of Five' and MCQs

Dr A J Hakim MA MRCP
Consultant Rheumatologist and General Physician
Whipp's Cross University Hospital
London

IMMUNOLOGY: 'BEST OF FIVE' QUESTIONS

For each of the questions select the ONE most appropriate answer from the options provided.

2.1   T cells commonly secrete which one of the following cytokines when stimulated?

- ☐   A   IL-1 and tumour necrosis factor beta (TNFβ)
- ☐   B   Interferon-beta (IFNβ)
- ☐   C   Interleukin-1 (IL-1) and interferon-beta (IFNβ)
- ☐   D   Interleukin-2 (IL-2) and interferon-gamma (IFNγ)
- ☐   E   Tumour necrosis factor alpha (TNFα)

2.2   In auto-immunity which one of the following pairings correctly matches cell type with site of immune surveillance?

- ☐   A   All of the options
- ☐   B   B-cell/bone marrow
- ☐   C   B-cell/thymus
- ☐   D   T-cell/bone marrow
- ☐   E   T-cell/spleen

2.3   Which one of the following immunodeficiency disorders is not associated with a primary B-cell abnormality?

- ☐   A   Common variable immunodeficiency
- ☐   B   Di George syndrome
- ☐   C   IgA deficiency
- ☐   D   Wiskott-Aldrich syndrome
- ☐   E   X-linked (Bruton's) agammaglobulinaemia

2.4   Type II cryoglobulinaemia is more often associated with which one of these conditions?

- ☐ A   Hepatitis C
- ☐ B   Multiple myeloma
- ☐ C   Rheumatoid arthritis
- ☐ D   Systemic lupus eythematosus
- ☐ E   Waldenström's macroglobulinaemia

2.5   A Fab fragment of an immunoglobulin constitutes which one of the following?

- ☐ A   The Fab portion of one heavy chain linked to one light chain
- ☐ B   The hypervariable region of the light and heavy chain
- ☐ C   The variable region of the light chain
- ☐ D   The variable region of the light chain
- ☐ E   Two Fab portions of one heavy chain linked to two light chains

IMMUNOLOGY: MULTIPLE CHOICE QUESTIONS

Mark your answers with a tick (True) or a cross (False) in the box provided.

2.6   Of the complement pathway

- ☐ A the liver is a site of complement component synthesis
- ☐ B factor B is cleaved by factor H forming a stable C3bBb complex in the 'alternative' pathway
- ☐ C the 'alternative' pathway positive-feedback loop is controlled by factor I
- ☐ D single IgG antibody-immune complex is the most efficient stimulant of the 'classical' pathway
- ☐ E C2 component deficiency is the most common isolated deficiency of complement among Caucasians

2.7   The following statements are correct:

- ☐ A IgA can activate complement via the alternative pathway
- ☐ B IgA normally represents less than 1% of the serum immunoglobulin pool
- ☐ C J-chains are associated with both IgA and IgM
- ☐ D the Fab fragment determines the class of immunoglobulin
- ☐ E IgE can cross the placenta

2.8   The following HLA associations are correct:

- ☐ A HLA DR3 and dermatitis herpetiformis
- ☐ B HLA A3 and schizophrenia
- ☐ C HLA DR2 and Goodpasture's syndrome
- ☐ D HLA DQW2 and coeliac disease
- ☐ E HLA DR7 and Hashimoto's thyroiditis

2.9   In the metabolism of arachidonic acid

☐ A   arachidonic acid is converted to leukotrienes via phospholipase A2

☐ B   corticosteroids inhibit phospholipase A2

☐ C   5-lipoxygenase is blocked by aspirin

☐ D   platelets are a major source of leukotrienes

☐ E   non-steroidal anti-inflammatory drugs with a high cyclo-oxygenase type 1 (COX 1) to type 2 (COX2) activity ratio may have fewer gastrointestinal side-effects

2.10   Activation of complement

☐ A   cannot occur without the participation of immunoglobulins

☐ B   results in increased capillary permeability

☐ C   protects cells from lysis by stabilising cell membranes

☐ D   does not occur in serum heated to 56c for 30 minutes

☐ E   leads to the migration of neutrophils into sites of inflammation

INFECTIOUS DISEASES

'Best of Five' and MCQs

Dr A J Hakim MA MRCP
Consultant Rheumatologist and General Physician
Whipp's Cross University Hospital
London

INFECTIOUS DISEASES: 'BEST OF FIVE' QUESTIONS

For each of the questions select the ONE most appropriate answer from the options provided.

3.1   **A 23-year-old male is investigated for hepatitis B virus (HBV) infection. Positive tests are found for hepatitis B surface antigen (HBsAg) and IgM antibodies to the core antigen (anti-HBc IgM) and a negative 'e' antigen (eAg). Which one of the following is the most likely clinical status?**

☐   A   Acute HBV infection

☐   B   Chronic HBV carrier

☐   C   Convalescence from acute HBV

☐   D   None of the options

☐   E   Previous immunization against HBV

3.2   **Which one of the following viral groups is least associated with haemorrhagic manifestations?**

☐   A   Arbovirus

☐   B   Arenavirus

☐   C   Paramyxovirus

☐   D   Picornavirus

☐   E   Rotavirus

3.3   **When comparing Rhodesian and Gambian sleeping sickness, which one of the following statements is not true of both conditions?**

☐   A   CNS abnormalities occur

☐   B   Hepatosplenomegaly occurs

☐   C   Humans are a recognised reservoir

☐   D   Melarsoprol is effective treatment

☐   E   The causative agent is *Trypanosoma brucei*

3.4 **In which one of the following malarial agents does a stage of exoerythrocytic schizogony definitely not occur?**

- ❑ E None of the options
- ❑ C *P. falciparum*
- ❑ B *P. malariae*
- ❑ D *P. ovale*
- ❑ A *P. vivax*

3.5 **A 43-year-old male African immigrant, recently arrived in the United Kingdom, is assessed by his general practitioner during registration. He has a long-standing right hemiplegia and is blind in his left eye. There is a history of recurrent pain and redness of the eyes with an occasional exudative discharge. The general practitioner notes several small hard subcutaneous nodules. Which one of the following is the most likely diagnosis?**

- ❑ A Cysticercosis
- ❑ B Filariasis
- ❑ C Hydatid disease
- ❑ D Schistosomiasis
- ❑ E Strongyloides

3.6 **All the following statements regarding Q fever are correct except one?**

- ❑ A Acute illness may resolve spontaneously without treatment
- ❑ B Osteomyelitis is a recognised complication
- ❑ C The causative agent is *Coxiella burnetii*
- ❑ D The Weil-Felix reaction is positive
- ❑ E Transmission of the disease to humans is independent of an arthropod vector

3.7 **Which one of the following is a high risk factor for contracting *Haemophilus*?**

- ❑ A Alcohol abuse
- ❑ B All of the options
- ❑ C Infancy and early childhood
- ❑ D Sickle cell disease
- ❑ E Splenectomy

3.8   A 40-year-old British abattoir worker becomes systemically ill with
        jaundice, microscopic haematuria and meningism. He is found to have mild
        renal impairment, and haemolytic anaemia. There is no rash, pharyngitis or
        lymphadenopathy. He has not travelled abroad. Which one of the following
        is the most probable diagnosis?

❏ A   Cholera

❏ B   Coxsackie virus A

❏ C   Infectious mononucleosis

❏ D   Leptospirosis

❏ E   Sporotrichosis

3.9   Which one of the following statements regarding staphylococcal and
        streptococcal infection is incorrect?

❏ A   Bacteraemia is uncommon in toxic shock syndrome

❏ B   Group A *Streptococcus* causes erysipelas

❏ C   Impetigo is associated with glomerulonephritis

❏ D   None of the options

❏ E   Scalded skin syndrome is caused by S. aureus

3.10   A leukaemic patient on chemotherapy presents with fever and a pulmonary
        infiltrate. Which one of the following infectious agents could present in this
        way?

❏ A   All of the options

❏ B   *Chlamydia*

❏ C   *Cryptococcus*

❏ D   Herpes simplex

❏ E   None of the options

3.11 A 26-year-old man with a history of injecting drugs is admitted with fever and malaise. His temperature is 39.3°C, pulse 126 beats/min and blood pressure 90/65 mmHg. He is mildly confused, but without symptoms of meningism or focal neurological signs. A loud murmur that increases with inspiration is audible at the lower left sternal edge. A plain chest radiograph shows several small cavitating lesions peripherally, but is otherwise normal. Which one of the following is the most likely diagnosis?

- ❑ A Acute HIV seroconversion illness
- ❑ B *Cryptococcus neoformans* infection
- ❑ C *Mycobacterium tuberculosis* infection
- ❑ D *Staphylococcus aureus* endocarditis and septicaemia
- ❑ E Tricuspid endocarditis due to *Streptococcus bovis*

3.12 Antibiotic chemotherapies employ several mechanisms of action. Some interfere with bacterial cell-wall synthesis and others penetrate well into cells and disrupt bacterial ribosomal function. Which one of the following drugs acts by interfering with ribosomal function?

- ❑ A Amoxycillin
- ❑ B Ciprofloxacin
- ❑ C Clarithromycin
- ❑ D Trimethoprim
- ❑ E Vancomycin

3.13 An 85-year-old Caucasian lady presents with fever, headache, neck stiffness and photophobia. She recently completed a three-day course of cefalexin for a urinary tract infection. Her past medical history is otherwise unremarkable. A lumbar puncture is performed and the cerebrospinal fluid (CSF) is found to be clear and colourless. The CSF biochemistry and microscopy shows a protein count of 1.7 g/l, a glucose of 3.1 mmol/l (plasma glucose 6.8 mmol/l), and a white cell count of 104 per mm^3 (lymphocytes 65%, polymorphs 35%). Occasional short Gram-positive rods are present. Which one of the following is the likely cause of her meningitis?

- ❑ A *Listeria monocytogenes*
- ❑ B *Mycobacterium tuberculosis*
- ❑ C *Neisseria meningitidis*
- ❑ D *Pseudomonas aeruginosa*
- ❑ E *Streptococcus pneumoniae*

3.14   Cytomegalovirus (CMV) is an important opportunistic infection in
         immunocompromised individuals. Of the five clinical complications of HIV-
         infection listed below, which one would be least likely to be due to CMV
         infection?

   ❏ A   Acalculous cholecystitis

   ❏ B   Encephalitis

   ❏ C   Nephritis

   ❏ D   Polyradiculopathy

   ❏ E   Retinitis

3.15   Which one of the following is a chemokine co-receptor that acts in
         conjunction with the CD4+ receptor to enable attachment of the HIV virus,
         membrane fusion, and internalisation of the contents of the HIV virus into
         the host cytoplasm?

   ❏ A   CCR5

   ❏ B   CD8+

   ❏ C   *Gp120*

   ❏ D   HIV protease enzyme

   ❏ E   pol gene product

3.16   A 35-year-old man presents with a two-day history of fever, malaise,
         wheeze, mild diarrhoea, an urticarial rash and hepatosplenomegaly. He
         recently returned from a three-month overland trip in East Africa. He can
         recall numerous insect bites on his trip and his adherence to anti-malarial
         prophylaxis has been poor. He swam in fresh water rivers and consumed
         local food and beverages. His full blood count on admission shows a
         normal haemoglobin and platelet count, but a raised white cell count of
         15.7 x 10^9/l (neutrophils 26%, lymphocytes 21%, eosinophils 45%,
         monocytes 1%). No malaria parasites are detected on three separate films.
         Which one of the following is the most likely diagnosis?

   ❏ A   Amoebiasis

   ❏ B   Dengue fever

   ❏ C   Leishmaniasis

   ❏ D   Malaria

   ❏ E   Schistosomiasis

3.17   A 43-year-old man, HIV-positive for 10 years, stopped all anti-retroviral
        treatments six months ago because of side-effects. His current CD4+ count
        is very low. Over the course of two months he has developed a hemiparesis
        and dysarthria, but has not been systemically unwell or febrile. A magnetic
        resonance (MRI) scan of the brain shows multiple cerebral white matter
        lesions that do not enhance with contrast or show mass effect. Cerebro-
        spinal fluid examination is within normal limits. Which one of the following
        organisms is most likely to be responsible for his symptoms?

    ❑   A   *Cryptococcus neoformans*
    ❑   B   JC virus
    ❑   C   *Mycobacterium tuberculosis*
    ❑   D   *Nocardia asteroides*
    ❑   E   *Toxoplasma gondii*

3.18   A 25-year-old woman is admitted to hospital acutely unwell with malaise,
        fever, profuse vomiting, and mild diarrhoea over a 36-hour period. There is
        no history of foreign travel and her food history is unremarkable. On
        admission her pulse is 130 beats/min, blood pressure 84/62 mmHg,
        temperature 38.9°C. She is confused, but has no focal neurology. She has a
        faint, erythematous rash, particularly noticeable on her extremities. Her
        tongue and buccal mucosa are noted to be red and hyperaemic. What is
        the most likely diagnosis?

    ❑   A   *E. coli* 0157 infection
    ❑   B   Meningococcal septicaemia
    ❑   C   *Salmonella* gastro-enteritis
    ❑   D   Toxic shock syndrome
    ❑   E   Typhoid fever

3.19   A 25-year-old man presents to a sexually transmitted diseases clinic. He
moved to the UK from West Africa four years ago. Five days ago he
developed a cluster of 10 small (1–2 mm), painful, punched-out ulcers on
the penis. The inguinal lymph nodes are tender and slightly enlarged, but
there is no evidence of suppuration. He has had unprotected sex with a
new partner recently. Which one of the following is the most likely
diagnosis?

- ❏   A   Behçet's disease
- ❏   B   Chancroid
- ❏   C   Genital herpes
- ❏   D   Lymphogranuloma venerum
- ❏   E   Syphilis

3.20   Which one of the following statements regarding anti-tuberculous
medication is incorrect?

- ❏   A   Capreomycin is ototoxic
- ❏   B   Macrolides may increase the risk of rifabutin-induced uveitis
- ❏   C   Rifampicin causes an orange discoloration of the urine and secretions
- ❏   D   Rifampicin is a potent liver enzyme inducer
- ❏   E   Toxic side-effects of isoniazid are best reduced by the concomitant use
of rifabutin

INFECTIOUS DISEASES: MULTIPLE CHOICE QUESTIONS

Mark your answers with a tick (True) or a cross (False) in the box provided.

3.21   The following statements are correct:

- [ ] A HIV infects lymphocytes via gp41 binding to the CD4 receptor
- [ ] B normal pathogens can behave opportunistically in HIV sero-positive patients when the CD4 count falls below 400
- [ ] C HIV can directly cause renal disease
- [ ] D hypogammaglobulinaemia is an expected complication of HIV infection
- [ ] E the action of reverse transcriptase leads to the synthesis of double-stranded DNA

3.22   In the biology of prion protein (PrP)

- [ ] A the protein can be inactivated by procedures that modify nucleic acids
- [ ] B PrP is encoded on the host genome
- [ ] C PrPc (cellular) human product has the same amino acid sequence as PrPsc (scrapie)
- [ ] D it is possible, in part, to determine the risk of early or late onset of disease by studying the genotype
- [ ] E MRI and cerebrospinal fluid protein analysis are diagnostic in Creutzfeldt–Jakob disease

3.23   The following vaccines are 'live-attenuated':

- [ ] A hepatitis A
- [ ] B influenza
- [ ] C pneumococcal
- [ ] D rabies
- [ ] E cholera

3.24   **The following conditions are 'notifiable' in the United Kingdom:**
- ☐ A   anthrax
- ☐ B   hepatitis A
- ☐ C   meningococcal meningitis
- ☐ D   poliomyelitis
- ☐ E   tuberculosis

3.25   **In schistosomiasis**
- ☐ A   eggs of *schistosoma* can be found in the urine
- ☐ B   seizures and hemiplegia may occur
- ☐ C   praziquantel is active against all types of schistosome
- ☐ D   cor-pulmonale is a recognised complication
- ☐ E   protective immunity follows infection

3.26   **In Rickettsial disease**
- ☐ A   the rash usually appears after 3 to 5 days of illness
- ☐ B   focal neurological symptoms are not a feature
- ☐ C   hepatic failure is common
- ☐ D   early acute serology is helpful
- ☐ E   chloramphenicol may be used in treatment

3.27   **Among the sexually transmitted diseases**
- ☐ A   the most common cause of non specific urethritis is gonococcus
- ☐ B   erythromycin is the treatment of choice for *Chlamydia*
- ☐ C   untreated non-specific urethritis has a very high risk of epididymitis and urethral strictures
- ☐ D   human papilloma virus types 16 and 18 are associated with cervical and anal malignancy
- ☐ E   most cases of pelvic inflammatory disease (PID) are caused by *N.gonorrhoea*

3.28   Insect borne infections include

- ☐ A   hanta virus
- ☐ B   dengue
- ☐ C   African trypanosomiasis
- ☐ D   marburg virus
- ☐ E   tularaemia

3.29   Of the protozoal infections

- ☐ A   pentavalent antimony compounds are the treatment of choice in trypanosomiasis
- ☐ B   the Paul Bunnell test is positive in toxoplasmosis
- ☐ C   amoebiasis is caused principally by *Entamoeba coli*
- ☐ D   the modified Ziehl–Neelson stain will identify cryptosporidia oocysts
- ☐ E   a negative stool examination excludes the diagnosis of giardiasis

3.30   In the treatment and complications of viral hepatitis

- ☐ A   high faecal shedding of hepatitis A occurs in the prodromal phase
- ☐ B   corticosteroids are indicated in acute disease
- ☐ C   acute hepatitis B can be differentiated from chronic disease by the presence of high Hbs Ag surface antigen titres
- ☐ D   chronic infection with hepatitis E increases the risk of hepatocellular carcinoma
- ☐ E   chronic hepatitis is the most common outcome of acute hepatitis C infection

3.31   Of the atypical pneumonias

- ☐ A   *Mycoplasma* are resistant to cell-wall active antibiotics
- ☐ B   *Mycoplasma* induced haemolytic anaemia is associated with cold agglutinin, anti I antibody formation
- ☐ C   *Mycoplasma* are Gram-positive on Gram stain smear
- ☐ D   Pontiac fever is an acute pneumonic form of legionellosis
- ☐ E   antibody based serological tests in legionella are highly specific

3.32   In brucellosis

☐   A   a leucocytosis is usual in acute infection

☐   B   the organism remains viable in dry soil

☐   C   freezing destroys the organism

☐   D   incidence is increasing in the United Kingdom

☐   E   organisms can be isolated from human breast milk

3.33   The following statements on fungal infections are true

☐   A   infection with *Coccidioides immitis* is usually mild or asymptomatic

☐   B   *Aspergillus* causes paranasal granulomas

☐   C   pneumonia is the commonest presentation of cryptococcosis

☐   D   serology is useful in confirming blastomycosis

☐   E   over 90% of endemic histoplasmosis infections are asymptomatic

3.34   In tuberculosis treatment

☐   A   isoniazid accelerates the metabolism of anti epileptics

☐   B   doses of oral hypoglycaemics may need to be increased during concomitant use of rifampicin

☐   C   streptomycin can cause ocular toxicity

☐   D   pyrazinamide may exacerbate acute gout

☐   E   drug induced hepatitis is typically chronic and unresolving

3.35   In the HIV sero-positive patient

☐   A   diarrhoea in the immunocompromised is most often caused by protozoal infection

☐   B   *Pneumocystis carinii* is a zoonosis

☐   C   *P. carinii* may appear as lobar consolidation on a chest radiograph

☐   D   tuberculosis can increase the load and spread of HIV

☐   E   central nervous system infection is a common early feature of disease

3.36   Amongst the complications of HIV and AIDS

☐ A   focal skin Kaposi sarcoma responds best to intralesional alpha-interferon

☐ B   large cell lymphomas are associated with Epstein–Barr virus (EBV)

☐ C   opportunistic infection of peripheral nerve and muscle is uncommon

☐ D   retinal microvascular cotton wool spots always require urgent treatment

☐ E   abdominal pain may be due to sclerosing cholangitis

3.37   Of the protozoal infections

☐ A   pentavalent antimony compounds are the treatment of choice in trypanosomiasis

☐ B   the Paul Bunnell test is positive in toxoplasmosis

☐ C   amoebiasis is caused principally by *Entamoeba coli*

☐ D   the modified Ziehl–Neelson stain will identify cryptosporidia oocysts

☐ E   a negative stool examination excludes the diagnosis of giardiasis

3.38   The following are causes of fever and pulmonary infiltrate in the immunocompromised:

☐ A   *Chlamydia*

☐ B   *Herpes simplex*

☐ C   cryptococcus

☐ D   nocardia

☐ E   candida

3.39   In *Plasmodium falciparum* malaria

☐ A   relapse from persistent liver infection is a feature

☐ B   parasites can synthesise pyrimidines *de novo*

☐ C   parasite specific G6PD may be found in host red blood cells

☐ D   primaquine is the drug of choice

☐ E   patients rarely present later than four weeks after returning from travel

3.40   **Features of borreliosis include**

☐   A   hepatic enlargement and tenderness

☐   B   petechial rash

☐   C   meningism

☐   D   myocarditis

☐   E   Jarisch–Herxheimer reaction

RHEUMATOLOGY

'Best of Five' and MCQs

Dr A J Hakim MA MRCP
Consultant Rheumatologist and General Physician
Whipp's Cross University Hospital
London

RHEUMATOLOGY: 'BEST OF FIVE' QUESTIONS

For each of the questions select the ONE most appropriate answer from the options provided.

4.1   A 50-year-old woman presents with knee pain. She is on medication for non-insulin-dependent diabetes mellitus, hypertension and moderate congestive cardiac failure. She has rheumatoid arthritis and is treated with methotrexate and low-dose prednisolone. She is commenced on a non-steroidal anti-inflammatory drug (NSAID). Which one of the following drugs can interact with the NSAID?

☐   A   Angiotensin converting enzyme inhibitors (ACE-I)

☐   B   Any of these items

☐   C   Methotrexate

☐   D   Oral hypogylcaemics

☐   E   Thiazide diuretics

4.2   A 72-year-old male presents to Accident and Emergency with a low-trauma fracture to the wrist following a seizure. He has taken phenytoin for seizures, a beta-blocker for hypertension, and prednisolone for polymyalgia rheumatica for many years. He complains of impotence and lethargy. In his history, which one of the following is not suggestive of a risk factor for osteoporosis?

☐   A   Being male and 72 years of age

☐   B   Impotence

☐   C   Use of a beta-blocker

☐   D   Use of corticosteroids

☐   E   Use of phenytoin

4.3 **Which one of the following statements regarding drug-induced lupus (DIL) is not true?**

☐ A Central nervous system and renal involvement is uncommon in DIL

☐ B Classical lupus skin findings (malar rash, oral ulcers, alopecia) are uncommon in DIL

☐ C Drugs implicated to cause DIL should not be used in idiopathic systemic lupus erythematosus

☐ D Methyldopa is implicated in causing DIL

☐ E More than 50% of patients taking procainamide for more than 12 months develop positive anti-nuclear antibody titres

4.4 **Anti-neutrophil cytoplasmic antibodies (ANCA) are associated with which one of the following?**

☐ A All of the following

☐ B Felty's syndrome

☐ C Human immunodeficiency virus

☐ D Inflammatory bowel disease

☐ E Wegener's granulomatosis

4.5 **A 24-year-old Iraqi male presents with recurrent attacks of generalised abdominal pain lasting up to 72 hours. He also describes a pleuritic-type pain, a swollen knee, and on more than one occasion has experienced a rash on his legs that is tender, swollen and well demarcated. Which one of the following statements is least likely to be true?**

☐ A A skin biopsy often demonstrates evidence of vasculitis

☐ B Fever is often a reported complaint

☐ C Persistent synovitis for more than a few months is uncommon

☐ D Proteinuria may be present

☐ E There is likely to be a leucocytosis

4.6 **The following are all diagnostic criteria for benign joint hypermobility syndrome except?**

- ☐ A Back pain
- ☐ B Beighton hypermobility score of 2 out of 9
- ☐ C Hernias
- ☐ D Joint pains in more than one joint for one week
- ☐ E Soft-tissue rheumatism in three or more sites

4.7 **Which one of the following statements regarding uric acid metabolism is incorrect?**

- ☐ A None of the following
- ☐ B Serum uric acid levels are increased in Fanconi's syndrome
- ☐ C Serum uric acid levels increase in metabolic acidosis
- ☐ D Spironolactone does not cause hyperuricaemia
- ☐ E Toxaemia of pregnancy is associated with increased purine turnover

4.8 **A 35-year-old woman is referred from her general practice following a presentation with shortness of breath, myalgia and arthralgia. Laboratory tests for extractable nuclear antigens are positive for anti-Sm, RNP, and Ro (SS-A). Which one of the following is the most likely diagnosis?**

- ☐ A Polymyositis
- ☐ B Rheumatoid arthritis
- ☐ C Sjögren's syndrome
- ☐ D Systemic lupus erythematosus
- ☐ E Systemic sclerosis

4.9 **Which one of the following is a feature of aggressive disease in rheumatoid arthritis?**

- ☐ A All of the options
- ☐ B Functional disability
- ☐ C High rheumatoid factor titre
- ☐ D Raised C-reactive protein
- ☐ E Rheumatoid nodules

4.10 A 58-year-old male presents with blurred vision, an occipital headache, fatigue and shoulder girdle pain. On examination he has scalp tenderness, myalgia but no myopathy, and no evidence of fundoscopic or neurological abnormality. Which one of the following would be the correct immediate action?

☐ A Commence a non-steroidal anti-inflammatory drug

☐ B Commence oral prednisolone at 20 mg/day

☐ C Request an ESR and temporal artery biopsy

☐ D Request a computerized tomography (CT) scan of the head

☐ E Start the patient on 60 mg/day oral prednisolone

4.11 A 34-year-old hiker returned from a two-week vacation in the American Great Lakes four weeks ago. He complains of a flitting arthralgia, myalgia, bone pain and a swollen knee. He recalls an episode lasting several days on vacation where he had a headache, irritated eyes, a sore throat and swollen glands, and he has a persistent rash. He denies sexual contact. Which one of the following would be the most useful diagnostic test?

☐ A Aspirate and culture the knee effusion for gonococcal infection

☐ B Biopsy the rash or a palpable lymph node

☐ C Measure serum anti-nuclear antibodies

☐ D Measure spirochaete antibodies

☐ E Measure the serum anti-streptolysin-O antibody titre (ASOT)

4.12 A 30-year-old woman collapses at her GP surgery. On arrival in A&E she is short of breath and hypoxic with pleuritic sounding chest pain. The patient is able to confirm she is already on warfarin following a similar episode a year ago and that she lost a pregnancy in the first three months just two years ago. There is a family history of arthritis and her sister takes medication for a kidney disease. Which one of the following statements is least correct in this scenario?

☐ A A ds-DNA antibody titre could be useful

☐ B Sudden widespread organ failure may occur

☐ C There is a risk of arterial as well as venous thrombosis

☐ D Thrombocytopenia may be present

☐ E Warfarin should be dosed to maintain the INR at 2.0

4.13 **Which one of the following is not a recognized cause of ectopic calcification or ossification of soft tissues?**

☐ A   Dermatomyositis

☐ B   Hyperparathyroidism

☐ C   Hypothyroidism

☐ D   Trauma

☐ E   Tumour lysis

4.14 **Pyoderma gangrenosum is not a feature of which one of the following rheumatic diseases?**

☐ A   Churg Strauss syndrome

☐ B   None of these

☐ C   Psoriatic arthritis

☐ D   Rheumatoid arthritis

☐ E   Wegener's granulomatosis

4.15 **A young man is diagnosed as having pseudohypoparathyroidism. Which one of the following laboratory tests is consistent with this diagnosis?**

☐ A   All of the following

☐ B   Hypercalcaemia

☐ C   Hypophosphataemia

☐ D   None of these items

☐ E   Raised parathyroid hormone

Rheumatology: 'Best of Five' Questions

Mark your answers with a tick (True) or a cross (False) in the box provided.

4.16   IgM rheumatoid factor

- ☐ A   indicates disease when present
- ☐ B   is not useful for monitoring treatment
- ☐ C   reacts with the Fc component of IgG
- ☐ D   is positive in infective endocarditis
- ☐ E   is positive in 50% of patients with rheumatoid nodules

4.17   Among the features of systemic lupus erythematosus

- ☐ A   joint disease is characteristically non-erosive
- ☐ B   Raynaud's disease is uncommon
- ☐ C   livedo reticularis is pathognomonic
- ☐ D   subacute cutaneous disease is usually benign
- ☐ E   hypertension is common

4.18   The following statements about the spondylo-arthropathies are correct:

- ☐ A   tissue typing for HLA-B27 is particularly useful
- ☐ B   they are more common in adult males
- ☐ C   transient disease is often non-erosive
- ☐ D   anterior uveitis occurs in 30% of patients
- ☐ E   sacro-iliitis can be unilateral or bilateral

4.19   Raynaud's phenomenon

- ☐ A   is much more common in women
- ☐ B   is a feature of Sjögren's syndrome
- ☐ C   can be treated with ACE-inhibitors
- ☐ D   is due to blood vessel hyper-reactivity
- ☐ E   affects 5–10% of the population

4.20   Features of Behçet's disease include

☐ A   central nervous system disorders

☐ B   erythema nodosum

☐ C   venous thrombosis in 75% of patients

☐ D   iritis

☐ E   diarrhoea

4.21   In septic arthritis

☐ A   a Gram stain should be done immediately

☐ B   turbidity of the aspirate implies infection

☐ C   clinical suspicion of Lyme disease would lead a clinician to chose tetracycline for 'blind' therapy

☐ D   rubella is accompanied by a self-limiting polyarthropathy

☐ E   beta haemolytic *Strep.* accounts for 50% of all cases

4.22   Sjögren's syndrome

☐ A   should be treated with topical steroid eye drops

☐ B   causes dyspareunia

☐ C   affects men more than women

☐ D   may cause facial swelling

☐ E   is associated with the Anti-SS-A antibody

4.23   In the crystal arthropathies

☐ A   acute gout is treated with uricosuric drugs

☐ B   blood urate is a reliable test for confirming gout

☐ C   all patients with hyperuricaemia should receive allopurinol

☐ D   hyperparathyroidism is associated with pseudo-gout

☐ E   the absence of chondrocalcinosis on X-ray rules out a diagnosis of pseudo-gout

4.24   Osteomalacia

- [ ] A   is associated with a myopathy
- [ ] B   causes reduced bone volume
- [ ] C   must be corrected by using the more potent forms of vitamin D such as 1-alpha hydroxycholecalciferol
- [ ] D   may result in tertiary hyperparathyroidism
- [ ] E   causes lesions that are undetectable on bone scintigraphy

4.25   In Paget's disease

- [ ] A   the alkaline phosphatase is always raised and a good marker of bone turnover
- [ ] B   the characteristic early lesion is a resorption front of abnormally large osteoclasts
- [ ] C   all bisphosphonates directly inhibit osteoblastic activity at therapeutic dose
- [ ] D   spread to other bones is a late feature of the disease
- [ ] E   paraparesis may occur

4.26   Reiter's syndrome

- [ ] A   is the most common cause of an inflammatory oligoarthropathy in young men
- [ ] B   is characterised by uveitis
- [ ] C   is associated with buccal ulceration
- [ ] D   is most often self limiting
- [ ] E   disease activity correlates well with the ESR

4.27   The causes of osteomalacia include

- [ ] A   primary biliary cirrhosis
- [ ] B   Fanconi syndrome
- [ ] C   acute renal failure
- [ ] D   renal tubular acidosis
- [ ] E   primary hyperparathyroidism

4.28   The following statements on osteogenesis imperfecta are correct:

☐   A   blue sclera are common to all types

☐   B   the condition is autosomal recessive

☐   C   hearing loss is mainly conductive

☐   D   aortic incompetence is a feature

☐   E   the biochemical disorder is of type II collagen

4.29   The following are secondary causes of osteoporosis:

☐   A   Klinefelter's syndrome

☐   B   Cushing's disease

☐   C   frusemide

☐   D   multiple myeloma

☐   E   acromegaly

4.30   The following are characteristic of polymyalgia rheumatica (PMR):

☐   A   depression

☐   B   weight loss

☐   C   lymphadenopathy

☐   D   raised muscle enzymes

☐   E   sternoclavicular joint swelling

CLINICAL PHARMACOLOGY: 'BEST OF FIVE' ANSWERS

1.1   B: Decrease in gut motility

Stimulation of the α-adrenoceptor leads to vasoconstriction of most vessels in the body, in particular in the skin, mucosae, abdominal viscera and coronary circulation. Further actions include decrease in gut motility, contraction of the pregnant uterus, decreased exocrine secretion by pancreatic acini and contraction of the radial muscle of the iris. Cholinergic activity and nitric oxide are largely responsible for penile erection.

1.2   C: Increased release of virus from cells

Zanamivir is a neuraminidase inhibitor, and is licensed for the treatment of influenza A or B within 48 hours of the onset of symptoms. Neuraminidase in the virus breaks down N-acetylneuraminic acid in respiratory secretions; this allows the virus to penetrate to the surfaces of cells. Inhibition of the neuraminidase prevents infection, and in some cases, complications such as otitis media. Neuraminidase is also necessary for the optimal release of virus from infected cells, an action that increases the spread of virus and the intensity of the infection. Inhibition of neuraminidase decreases the likelihood of illness and reduces the severity of any illness that does develop. Zanamivir is inhaled through the mouth; the majority of the drug ends up in the oropharynx; overall, the drug is only 10–20% bioavailable. Zanamivir can decrease bronchial airflow, and should be used with caution in patients with chronic respiratory disease in whom it can induce clinically significant bronchospasm.

1.3   B: Can cause neutropenia and thrombocytopenia

Cephalosporins, like the penicillins, have a β-lactam ring. There is therefore a 20% risk of cross-sensitivity between the two groups; if a patient has had a severe reaction to penicillin such as anaphylaxis, then cephalosporin should either not be used at all or with extreme caution. Most cephalosporins have half-lives less than 3 hours. Cephalosporins are associated with a number of adverse effects including skin rashes, anaphylaxis, neutropenia and thrombocytopenia, and are one of the most important causes of *Clostridium difficile* diarrhoea. Indeed, the current epidemic of *Clostridium difficile* diarrhoea has been blamed on the British Thoracic Society guidelines that recommended the use of cephalosporins in the treatment of community-acquired pneumonia.

1.4   D: Sarcoidosis

The hypercalcaemia of sarcoidosis responds to steroids better than the other causes listed. Irrespective of the cause of hypercalcaemia, the first choice of treatment should always be rehydration with normal saline. Frusemide used concomitantly does not provide a better calcium reducing effect. Only when patients have been rehydrated should bisphosphonates be used.

1.5   A: Approximately 8% of the population cannot convert codeine to morphine

Morphine is the drug of choice for controlling severe forms of pain. It is available in various formulations including:

- Normal release: onset of action 20 min; peak drug levels 60 min.

- Twice daily controlled release preparations: onset of action 1–2 hours; peak drug levels at 4 hours.

- Once daily controlled release preparation: slower onset of action with peak drug levels at 8.5 hours.

Both diamorphine and codeine are pro-drugs being converted to morphine in the body. Diamorphine is more soluble than morphine. Codeine is converted to morphine by the P450 enzyme CYP2D6, which is polymorphically expressed, being absent in 8–10% of the population. Many of the effects of morphine are subject to the phenomenon of tolerance including the analgesic and euphoric effects. Importantly, miosis is not subject to tolerance and can be used as a sign to indicate opiate misuse.

1.6   C: Drugs with intrinsic sympathomimetic activity are less likely to cause bradycardia

β-blockers have many different properties, which can be used to differentiate their actions and side-effect profile. These include lipophilicity, cardioselectivity and intrinsic sympathomimetic activity (ISA). β-blockers with ISA are less likely to cause bradycardia. β-blockers such as atenolol are cardio-selective but not cardio-specific; this means that they can still affect β_2 receptors especially when used in high dosage. β-blockers have class II antiarrhythmic properties and apart from sotalol (which also has class III properties) are unlikely to affect the Q-T interval. Celiprolol is a 'vasodilating' β-blocker and usually decreases total peripheral resistance. Esmolol is a short-acting β-blocker that is given intravenously to treat supraventricular arrhythmias.

1.7   A: Can cause selective IgA deficiency

Phenytoin is an anticonvulsant used for the treatment of generalised tonic clonic
convulsions and partial seizures. It can worsen myoclonic epilepsy, and can
precipitate seizures when levels are high. It displays zero order kinetics, i.e. due
to saturation of metabolism; small changes in dose can lead to disproportionate
increase in serum levels, with dose-dependent toxicity. It can cause a wide variety
of adverse effects including immune-mediated adverse reactions such as skin
rashes, hepatitis and aplastic anaemia. It can also lead to other immunological
abnormalities affecting both the cellular and humoral arms of the immune system.
With respect to the latter, selective IgA deficiency is a well-recognised adverse
reaction. Phenytoin is an enzyme inducer and can cause vitamin D deficiency,
leading to osteomalacia. Phenytoin is also an antiarrhythmic used to treat digoxin-
induced arrhythmias. It can however also lead to rhythm abnormalities such as
bradycardia and ectopic beats in 2% of patients.

1.8   A: Cimetidine and dapsone

Rifampicin is an enzyme inducer, which can lower cyclosporin levels leading to
graft rejection. This is a serious interaction that can be overcome by monitoring
cyclosporin levels and increasing the dose.

Cimetidine is an enzyme inhibitor that can inhibit phenytoin metabolism, leading
to phenytoin toxicity.

Ritonavir is a potent enzyme inhibitor; it can inhibit the metabolism of fluoxetine,
which can lead to a potentially fatal reaction called the serotonin syndrome.

Erythromycin is an enzyme inhibitor that can affect the metabolism of cisapride;
this can lead to prolongation of the Q-T interval and occasionally to torsade de
pointes and sudden death.

Cimetidine is an enzyme inhibitor, which is known to inhibit dapsone metabolism.
However, it results in reduced formation of a toxic metabolite of dapsone; this
toxic metabolite is known to cause methaemoglobinaemia. This combination has
therefore been used in patients with dermatitis herpetiformis to improve the
tolerability of dapsone.

1.9   A: Blood glucose > 8.3 mmol/l

Iron overdose is more common in children than in adults. Severe poisoning is characterised by haematemesis, hypotension, coma and shock. Disintegrating tablets may make the stools grey or black in colour, and this does not necessarily indicate a gastro-intestinal bleed. A white cell count of $> 15 \times 10^9/l$ and blood glucose level > 8.3 mmol/l in the six hours after ingestion, together with the presence of tablets on abdominal X-ray, have been shown to correlate with serum iron concentrations > 54 mmol/l. A challenge dose of desferrioxamine, if it results in urine with a red/orange colour, indicates the presence of free circulating iron, and is an indication for further treatment with desferrioxamine.

1.10   D: Rivastigmine binds to both the anionic and esteratic sites of the enzyme

Alzheimer's disease is characterised by decreased acetylcholine activity, and currently available drugs aim to increase cholinergic activity. Acetylcholine is broken down by acetylcholinesterase (AChE), and inhibition will increase acetylcholine activity. Acetylcholinesterase has both anionic and esteratic sites; its activity can be inhibited by binding to either site. Tacrine and donepezil act at the anionic site in a reversible fashion; they thus have a relatively short duration of enzyme inhibition. However, donepezil has a long half-life (70 hours) and thus only needs to be dosed once daily. Metrifonate is a pro-drug, which is converted to an active metabolite that binds irreversibly to the esteratic site of AChE. Like acetylcholine, rivastigmine binds to both the anionic and esteratic sites; it needs to be administered twice daily.

1.11   E: Vigabatrin – anterior uveitis

Cerivastatin is an HMG-CoA reductase inhibitor that is highly potent, but causes rhabdomyolysis to a greater extent than the other HMG-CoA reductase inhibitors. Indinavir is a protease inhibitor that can crystallise out in urine particularly when concentrations in plasma are high, and may in some cases lead to renal stones. Tolcapone is a COMT inhibitor used in Parkinson's disease; it was withdrawn because of its potential to cause hepatotoxicity and neuroleptic malignant syndrome. Vigabatrin causes peripheral visual field constriction in 30% of patients; this is thought to be irreversible, and although the mechanism of the adverse effect is not known, the retina is thought to be the site of toxicity. Pergolide is a dopamine agonist, and like all drugs of this class, it can cause fibrotic reactions including pulmonary fibrosis, pleural fibrosis and retroperitoneal fibrosis.

1.12   E: It inhibits purine synthesis

Leflunomide is a disease-modifying anti-rheumatic drug, like gold, penicillamine, chloroquine, cyclosporin, sulfasalazine, methotrexate, and azathioprine. Leflunomide inhibits pyrimidine synthesis through inhibition of dihydroorotate dehydrogenase, and is rapidly converted to an active metabolite. Its efficacy is comparable to that of sulfasalazine and methotrexate.

1.13   B: Dose requirements are genetically determined

Warfarin is an oral anticoagulant, which acts as a vitamin K antagonist by inhibiting vitamin K epoxide reductase. Dose requirements vary widely; these are at least partly determined by genetic polymorphisms affecting the P450 enzymes (CYP2C9) responsible for the metabolism of warfarin. The dose can be adjusted by monitoring the international normalised ratio (INR). Overdosage predisposes to bleeding, which can be treated with fresh frozen plasma and vitamin K. Warfarin does not affect bone density; however, osteoporosis can be caused by heparin.

1.14   A: Accidental injection of lignocaine into the systemic circulation may increase myocardial and neuronal excitability

Lignocaine, an amide local anaesthetic, is commonly used for minor surgery and in dental practice. Its duration of action can be prolonged by the addition of adrenaline, which causes vasoconstriction. Lignocaine is shorter acting than bupivacaine, and undergoes extensive metabolism. Intravenous injection can lead to cardiac arrhythmias and seizures.

1.15   D: The incidence of benign breast disease may be increased

Oral contraceptives contain progestogens, which inhibit LH release, while the oestrogen component inhibits FSH release. Oestrogens particularly at high dosage promote blood clotting; this risk is increased in women over 35 years, who are obese and smokers. Third generation oral contraceptives have a 2-fold higher risk of venous thromboembolism than second generation compounds. Thrombogenicity is also increased in patients who are carriers of the Factor V Leiden mutation. There is also a small increase in the absolute risk of stroke with the oral contraceptive. The oral contraceptive pill also has many beneficial effects including a reduced risk of benign breast disease and ovarian cancer.

1.16   A: Does not have a beneficial effect if administered at the time of the first ever demyelinating event

Interferon-beta has demonstrated benefits in the treatment of patients with established multiple sclerosis, including slowing the progression of physical disability, reducing the rate of clinical relapses, and reducing the development of brain lesions, as assessed by MRI, and brain atrophy. A recent study has shown that initiating treatment at the time of the first demyelinating event is beneficial in patients with lesions on MRI that indicate a high risk of clinically definite multiple sclerosis.

1.17   E: Trazodone

Drug	Anticholinergic	Cardiac	Nausea effects	Sedation effects
Amitriptyline	+++	+++	+	+++
Clomipramine	+++	++	+	++
Dothiepin	++	++	-	+++
Lofepramine	++	+	+	+
Trazodone	+	+	++	++

1.18   D: It inhibits the release of calcitonin gene-related peptide

Sumatriptan does not affect the aura of migraine and should be taken as soon as the headache starts. Triptans exhibit highly selective and potent agonist activity at the 1B, 1D, 1F and 1A 5HT receptors. Stimulation of the 5-HT_{1D} receptor inhibits CGRP release and thus dural vasodilatation. Sumatriptan should not be used in patients with ischaemic heart disease, Prinzmetal's angina and severe systemic hypertension. It should not be used with ergotamine, which can also cause coronary vasoconstriction. The drug is almost 100% bioavailable after subcutaneous administration, while bioavailability after oral administration is 14%.

1.19   B: it is a selective inhibitor of the neuronal uptake of noradrenaline

Bupropion (zyban) was initially used as an antidepressant, but has recently been licensed for smoking cessation. It inhibits the uptake of both noradrenaline and serotonin; it reduces nicotine craving and withdrawal symptoms. Patients treated with bupropion are twice as likely to have stopped smoking at 1 year compared to those on nicotine replacement therapy. Bupropion is associated with a large number of adverse effects; seizures occur in 1/1000 patients, while skin rashes are common, with a small number getting Stevens-Johnson syndrome. Bupropion is metabolised by a P450 enzyme called CYP2B6, but inhibits another P450 enzyme called CYP2D6, and can therefore be involved in interactions.

1.20   D: Oxcarbazepine

Hyoscine, neostigmine, codeine and propranolol are present in milk in concentrations that are too low to have a significant effect on the infant. Of the β-blockers, most are excreted in too small amounts to have an effect, but the infant should be monitored for bradycardia. Acebutolol, atenolol, nadolol and sotalol are present in greater amounts than other β-blockers. Appendix 5 of the BNF is a good source of information on drugs excreted in breast milk.

1.21   E: Vincristine

Vincristine is a vinca alkaloid treatment; it has no role in the treatment of minimal change glomerulonephritis. Nephrotic syndrome due to minimal change nephropathy is responsive to all the other agents.

1.22   A: Analgesic nephropathy was previously the commonest cause of renal failure in Australia

Analgesic nephropathy virtually always occurs after a cumulative dose of analgesics of at least 1 kg. It does not usually occur until heavy use has taken place for two years. Between 1950 and 1970, analgesic nephropathy was the commonest cause of renal failure in Australia, but has waned since phenacetin was banned. The primary renal lesion is papillary necrosis, which can also be caused by other aetiologies (e.g. diabetes, urinary obstruction, and sickle cell disease). Many patients have been successfully transplanted.

1.23   C: Analgesic nephropathy is characterised pathologically by glomerulonephritis

The renal lesion of analgesic nephropathy is papillary necrosis. Amphotericin B reduces renal blood flow and causes renal tubular acidosis.

1.24   A: Concomitant administration of diuretics makes aminoglycoside toxicity more likely

Toxicity may be avoided by dose reduction or reduced dosage frequency. Aminoglycosides require peak and trough levels for accurate estimation of potential nephrotoxicity. Aminoglycoside toxicity is more likely in a dehydrated patient or in the presence of hypokalaemia. Vancomycin is cleared renally and with renal impairment, therapeutic levels can be found up to five days after a single dose; drug levels should guide further doses. All drugs reach steady state after 5 half lives.

1.25   C: Nifedipine

Cholestyramine is an ion exchange resin used in the management of hypercholesterolaemia. As it is not absorbed, GI side-effects are common, particularly constipation. The commonest side-effect of verapamil therapy is constipation. Nifedipine affects different calcium channels from those affected by verapamil, and in particular does not affect the channels in the large bowel to the same extent. TCA and disopyramide have anticholinergic side-effects including constipation. Thiazides may cause constipation indirectly by hypercalcaemia, hypokalaemia or by dehydration.

1.26   B: Glypressin

Intravenous ranitidine is of no value in GI haemorrhage due to varices. Antibiotics reduce mortality in these patients presenting for the first time. Octreotide reduces the risk of rebleeding, but not mortality. Propranolol is most effective for prevention of rebleeding.

1.27   A: Digoxin

Metformin is normally inactivated in the liver and should be avoided because it causes lactic acidosis. Erythromycin is associated with a risk of hepatotoxicity and should be avoided in liver failure. Digoxin is excreted unchanged by the kidneys. Propranolol undergoes extensive first pass metabolism and this will not occur in liver disease, thus increasing the systemic availability. All opiates should be avoided because of the increased risk of coma.

1.28   A: Acute alcohol intake

Paracetamol is metabolised to a quinone-amine metabolite which is normally conjugated with glutathione. In paracetamol overdose, glutathione is depleted and the metabolite induces liver necrosis. Patients with reduced stores of glutathione are at increased risk of paracetamol toxicity, (e.g. malnourished, patients with anorexia and HIV positive patients). Increased production of the toxic metabolite will also increase the risk of toxicity, e.g. patients on enzyme inducers such as phenytoin, carbamazepine and rifampicin. Isoniazid is known to be an enzyme inhibitor and inducer and has been shown to increase risk of paracetamol toxicity. Acute alcohol intake is an enzyme inhibitor as opposed to chronic alcohol intake which is an enzyme inducer. Despite this, it would be unwise to treat patients with a history of acute alcohol intake as low risk and many of these have a history of chronic alcohol abuse.

1.29   E: Reducing nucleotide biosynthesis

Methotrexate binds to the intracellular enzyme dihydrofolate reductase. This enzyme is responsible for the production of reduced dihydrofolate, which is a co-factor involved in the synthesis of nucleotides and the amino acids serine and methionine. Methotrexate therefore interferes with nucleotide and protein synthesis. Methotrexate can be given orally or intravenously. Folinic acid is often given 24 hours after high-dose intravenous methotrexate treatment. This helps reduce the severity of methotrexate-induced myelosuppression and mucositis.

1.30   B: Busulphan

Other cytotoxic drugs that can cause lung fibrosis include bleomycin and methotrexate. These drugs cause acute interstitial pulmonary inflammation, that result in fibrotic changes. The diagnosis of drug-induced lung fibrosis is suggested by bilateral CXR shadowing in conjunction with a restrictive defect on pulmonary function testing. The differential diagnosis in cancer patients receiving chemotherapy is of metastatic carcinoma or pulmonary infection (often atypical). The diagnosis of lung fibrosis is confirmed by high resolution CT scanning (which typically shows fibrosis and ground glass appearance, the latter indicating active inflammation) and bronchoscopy with trans-bronchial biopsy for histological examination (or biopsy by video-assisted thoracoscopy).

1.31   C: The G1 and S phases

The stages of the cell cycle begin with the G0 (latent) phase. G1 is the resting phase when the cellular components required for DNA are synthesized. Cells then enter the S phase when DNA is synthesized. Then there is the G2 (pre-mitotic) phase, leading to the M (mitosis) phase. 5-Fluorouracil inhibits the synthesis of nucleotides during late G1, so preventing the synthesis of DNA during the S phase.

1.32   D: Chronic myeloid leukaemia

Hydroxyurea is an analogue of urea. It reduces the activity of the enzyme ribonucleotide reductase, which results in the inhibition of DNA synthesis. It is mainly used in the treatment of patients with chronic myeloid leukaemia who do not receive aggressive chemotherapy regimes or bone marrow transplantation. It is administered orally. High doses may cause gastrointestinal side-effects (e.g. nausea, vomiting and diarrhoea). Bone marrow suppression is another possible side-effect.

1.33   B: Dapsone

Rifampicin, sulfonamides, griseofulvin, and chloroquine should not be used in people with acute intermittent porphria (autosomal dominant inheritance). Penicillins, tetracyclines and chloramphenicol are safe to use.

1.34   D: Metformin

Insulin resistance is a state in which normal concentrations of insulin produce a subnormal biological response. Patients with insulin resistance have hyper-insulinaemia together with normoglycaemia or hyperglycaemia. It is commonly associated with obesity, non-insulin dependent diabetes mellitus, and essential hypertension. The insulin resistance syndrome includes impaired insulin stimulated glucose uptake, hyperinsulinaemia, glucose intolerance, hypertension, and dyslipidaemia. Drugs such as corticosteroids, β-blockers, and high dose thiazides can exacerbate insulin resistance; angiotensin converting enzyme inhibitors and α-blockers may reduce the resistance. Other factors which can improve insulin resistance include optimizing weight, aerobic exercise, stopping smoking, and moderate alcohol consumption. Metformin improves multiple aspects of the insulin resistance syndrome. Novel insulin enhancing drugs including thiazolidinediones are under evaluation.

1.35   D: Reduces the risk of vertebral fractures by 30%

Raloxifene, a Selective Estrogen Receptor Modulator (SERM), is a non-steroidal benzothiophene chemically related to tamoxifen. It is extensively glucuronidated in the gut wall and liver, with a mean bioavailability of the active drug of 2%. Plasma concentrations peak 6 hours after an oral dose and an elimination half-life of around 28 hours allows once-daily dosing. Excretion of raloxifene and its metabolites is mainly in the faeces, with less than 6% appearing in the urine. It is currently used for the prevention of non-traumatic vertebral fractures in postmenopausal women considered at increased risk of osteoporosis. It has been shown to reduce the risk of vertebral body fractures by 30%, although it has had no impact in reducing the rate of non-vertebral body fractures. It does not result in post-menopausal vaginal bleeding and reduces the risk of developing breast carcinoma. It does not reduce menopausal vasomotor symptoms. Other side-effects include venous thromboembolism, thrombophlebitis, hot flushes, leg cramps and peripheral oedema.

1.36   C: Captopril

In patients with uncomplicated diabetes, hypertension may be treated initially with a low dose of a thiazide diuretic (e.g. 2.5mg bendrofluazide daily) – in higher doses thiazides can exacerbate hyperglycaemia and dyslipidaemia. A cardio-selective β-blocker such as atenolol is an alternative but can interfere with awareness of hypoglycaemia. If these fail to lower blood pressure, or if unwanted effects occur, an ACE inhibitor, calcium channel blocker or α-blocker can be tried. In hypertensive patients with **diabetic nephropathy** blood pressure reduction slows the decline in renal function and ACE inhibitors are the treatment of choice, being more effective in this respect than other antihypertensive drugs.

CLINICAL PHARMACOLOGY: MULTIPLE CHOICE ANSWERS

1.37   A D

The mode of action of antibiotics can be classified as follows:

a) Inhibition of bacterial cell wall synthesis: penicillins, cephalosporins, vancomycin and teicoplanin

b) Inhibition of cell membrane synthesis: lincomycins

c) Inhibition of protein synthesis: aminoglycosides, tetracycline, macrolides, chloramphenicol and clindamycin

d) Inhibition of DNA synthesis: rifampicin, quinolone antibiotics, metronidazole, sulphonamides and trimethoprim.

1.38   A

In patients with IDDM, effective control of blood sugar has been shown to decrease long-term complications responsible for the morbidity and mortality of the disease. During an intercurrent infection, patients should not reduce insulin dosage as this may lead to diabetic ketoacidosis. Human insulin is now the most widely used form of insulin although some patients still use animal insulin. In theory, human insulin should be less immunogenic than porcine insulin, although this has not been borne out in clinical trials. Insulin lispro is an insulin analogue which is more rapidly absorbed; peak concentrations in blood occur earlier and loss from circulation is more rapid. Insulin lispro therefore has a more rapid onset of action, and postprandial glucose concentrations do not rise as high as with soluble insulin, and mild hypoglycaemia may be less common. Glycosylated haemoglobin (HbA1$_c$) does not change very much with insulin lispro, possibly because blood glucose before the next meal tends to be higher than with soluble insulin.

1.39   A C D

Tamoxifen is a partial agonist of the oestrogen receptor. It behaves as an oestrogen antagonist in breast tissue but has weak agonist effects on the endometrium, bone remodelling and cholesterol metabolism. The drug's main use is in breast cancer where it is more effective in postmenopausal women than in premenopausal women. It is currently being tested to determine whether it prevents the development of breast cancer in women with a positive family history. Because of its partial agonist activity, it can lead to the development of endometrial cancer and hypercalcaemia in patients with bony metastases. Tamoxifen also causes retinopathy.

1.40   B C D E

Protease inhibitors inhibit the viral aspartyl protease. They have largely been used in combination with two nucleoside analogues: such regimens have been shown to retard disease progression and decrease mortality. Resistance to protease inhibitors has been reported and is more likely to occur in patients with low blood levels, thus the importance of complying with therapy. Protease inhibitors also inhibit the cytochrome P450 enzymes and can therefore be responsible for clinically significant drug interactions with compounds such as midazolam (excess sedation) and rifabutin (uveitis). They have recently been reported to cause peripheral lipodystrophy which is characterised by fat re-distribution, hypertension, hyperglycaemia, insulin resistance, and possibly accelerated atherosclerosis. In light of this novel form of toxicity, their benefit-risk ratio needs to be re-evaluated.

1.41   B C

Warfarin is associated with skeletal and CNS defects if the foetus is exposed in the first trimester, while exposure during the third trimester increases the risk of intracranial haemorrhage during delivery. Misoprostol is associated with the Moebius sequence. Diazepam, oral contraceptives and aspirin were initially thought to possess some teratogenic risk, but formal cohort and case-control studies, and meta-analyses, have provided some evidence that these drugs are safe.

1.42   A B C D

Oestrogens should be combined with progestogens in patients with an intact uterus to reduce the risk of endometrial cancer. HRT has many benefits including prevention of bone loss, ischaemic heart disease and dementia, and the relief of menopausal symptoms. There are also many risks, including an increased risk of endometrial cancer (even in patients taking combined hormone therapy), breast cancer and venous thromboembolism. The beneficial effect of HRT on bone loss is more marked in patients who begin therapy within the five years after the menopause. Raloxifene is a new non-steroidal selective estrogen receptor modulator (SERM). It has oestrogenic effects on bone and serum lipids, but does not stimulate endometrial growth (i.e. it exerts an anti-oestrogenic effect). Preliminary findings suggest that it is also protective against breast cancer.

1.43   C E

Gastric lavage is best reserved for patients who present within two hours of an overdose, although with drugs that reduce gastric emptying, for example, anticholinergics, the time interval can be longer. Ipecacuanha syrup is associated with an increased risk of aspiration pneumonitis and oesophageal damage, and should not be used. Haemodialysis is useful for drugs with a low volume of distribution (i.e. drugs such as aspirin which reside mostly within the plasma) and is not used for drugs with a high volume of distribution, such as tricyclic antidepressants.

1.44   A B D

Grapefruit juice contains compounds that are inhibitors of the cytochrome P450 isoform CYP3A4. The ability of grapefruit juice to inhibit drug metabolism was first shown with the calcium channel blocker felodipine. Subsequent investigations have shown that grapefruit juice can interact with many CYP3A4 substrates including terfenadine (leading to Q-T prolongation), cisapride (Q-T prolongation), cyclosporin (cyclosporin toxicity), and the protease inhibitors. The interaction with the protease inhibitors can in fact be used therapeutically to increase their bioavailability, and thus their effectiveness.

1.45   B C E

Drug metabolism is conventionally divided into two phases, phase I and phase II. The main role of drug metabolism is to convert lipophilic compounds into hydrophilic metabolites, which can then be excreted from the body. Drug metabolism can also result in the formation of toxic metabolites that may be responsible for idiosyncratic toxicity. Phase I pathways are usually catalysed by cytochrome P450 enzymes, of which there are many different isoforms, while phase II pathways are catalysed by a number of enzymes including glucuronyl transferase and N-acetyl transferase. Many of these enzymes can be either inhibited or induced, and some also show genetically determined deficiencies. Metabolism occurs in all organs apart from those of ectodermal origin. The liver is the main site; other sites include skin, gut wall, kidney, lungs and brain.

1.46   A

Typical neuroleptic drugs such as chlorpromazine have been used for many years in the treatment of schizophrenia. Their usefulness is limited by their propensity to cause extrapyramidal adverse effects. Atypical neuroleptics are less likely to cause extrapyramidal adverse effects. Additionally, they affect not only the positive symptoms (like the typical neuroleptics), but also affect the negative symptoms, which are not improved by the typical neuroleptics. In comparison with the typical neuroleptics, the atypical neuroleptics are less likely to cause neuroleptic malignant syndrome and hyperprolactinaemia (except perhaps risperidone), but are more likely to induce weight gain. Atypical neuroleptics include clozapine, risperidone, olanzapine, sertindole, and quetiapine.

1.47   C D

Anticonvulsants often have more than one mode of action, although their efficacy can often be rationalised on the basis of one main mode of action. In general, the mode of action of anticonvulsants can be divided into one of three groups.

a) Inhibition of sodium conductance: these include phenytoin, carbamazepine, sodium valproate and lamotrigine.

b) Enhancement of GABAergic action in the CNS: this may be secondary to binding to the GABA receptor (phenobarbitone, benzodiazepines), inhibition of GABA transaminase (vigabatrin) and inhibition of GABA re-uptake (tiagabine).

c) Miscellaneous: includes inhibition of calcium conductance (ethosuximide) and drugs such as gabapentin where the mode of action has not yet been determined.

1.48   B C E

Lithium is used for bipolar (treatment and prophylaxis) and unipolar (prophylaxis) depression. It does not affect mood in normal individuals. It is handled like sodium by the body and is excreted via the kidneys. Therefore, its use should be avoided in patients with moderate to severe renal impairment. It is also excreted in breast milk and its use should be avoided in breast-feeding mothers. It has a narrow therapeutic index, and its levels need to be monitored. Its renal excretion can be affected by NSAIDs and diuretics, which can precipitate lithium toxicity. Adverse effects include goitre, hypothyroidism, tremor, convulsions and nephrogenic diabetes insipidus.

1.49   A B D E

An acute attack of gout should be treated with high-dose NSAIDs or colchicine. Commencement of therapy for chronic gout with drugs such as allopurinol or uricosurics such as probenecid, if not covered by NSAIDs, can sometimes precipitate an acute attack. Aspirin and salicylates antagonise the uricosuric drugs and therefore should be avoided in patients with gout. Other drugs that can cause hyperuricaemia include diuretics, adenosine, cyclosporin, inosine pranobex and alcohol.

1.50   A C D E

Clindamycin penetrates bone well and is active against *Staphylococcus aureus*, and thus can be used in the treatment of osteomyelitis. It is particularly liable to cause pseudomembranous colitis. Methicillin-resistant *S. aureus* (MRSA or 'superbugs') have attracted media attention recently. In most cases, it can be eliminated by topical therapy. Systemic therapy is only required when systemic infection is suspected: teicoplanin may be effective in such cases. Co-amoxiclav can cause cholestatic hepatitis which can appear up to six weeks after stopping the drug. The liver toxicity is thought to be due to clavulanic acid rather than amoxycillin. Clarithromycin, a macrolide, is often used in HIV-positive patients for prophylaxis against atypical mycobacteria.

1.51   A E

Manufacturers of generic drugs are required by law to show that their drug is bioequivalent to the brand leader. That is, the generic drug must be absorbed at the same rate and to the same extent as the brand leader. A drug can be categorised as being bioequivalent if it is shown that the absorption is within ± 20% of the branded product. The specified range is narrower for drugs such as warfarin which have a narrow therapeutic index. Bioequivalent studies are usually performed in volunteers and are single-dose studies. Bioequivalence is difficult to demonstrate with modified-release preparations, which should be prescribed by brand name. Different brands of drugs such as lithium and cyclosporin vary widely in bioavailability and should also be prescribed by brand name.

1.52   B C E

A first-pass effect means that the drug is extensively metabolised before it reaches the systemic circulation. Thus, drugs with a high first-pass effect have low bioavailability. Most drugs exhibit first-order kinetics; some drugs exhibit zero-order kinetics which means that there may be a disproportionate increase in serum concentration for a small increment in dose. The terminal half-life of a drug refers to the time required to excrete half of a given dose. Glucuronidation increases the water solubility of a drug.

1.53   A D

Digoxin is a narrow therapeutic index drug. Toxicity (even when levels are within the therapeutic range) can be precipitated by hypokalaemia, hypomagnesaemia and hypercalcaemia. Changes in the plasma sodium concentration have no effect on digoxin toxicity *per se*. Digoxin toxicity may manifest with symptoms such as nausea, vomiting, xanthopsia or ECG changes such as S-T depression (reversed tick pattern) or cardiac arrhythmias. Phenytoin can be used to treat digoxin-induced cardiac arrhythmias.

1.54   B D

The cause of motor neurone disease (MND) is unknown. It has been postulated that excitotoxic neurotransmitters such as glutamate may be involved in the pathogenesis of MND. Riluzole antagonises the effects of glutamate on nerve cells by inhibiting its release and protecting cells from glutamate-mediated damage. It has been licensed 'to extend life or the time to mechanical ventilation for patients with amyotrophic lateral sclerosis'. It is not licensed for use in other forms of MND such as progressive muscular atrophy or progressive bulbar palsy. Riluzole has a modest effect on mortality in patients with amyotrophic lateral sclerosis, but there is no evidence that it improves either functional capacity or quality of life. Riluzole causes an elevation of liver enzymes in more than 1% of patients.

1.55   A B C E

Drugs can cause anaemia by various mechanisms:

a) increased blood loss from the gastro-intestinal tract: aspirin, NSAIDs, meloxicam and alendronate;

b) increased red cell breakdown secondary to haemolysis: this may be metabolic (e.g. G6PD deficiency) or autoimmune (nomifensine, methyldopa);

c) deficiency of vitamin B_{12} or folic acid leading to megaloblastic anaemia: metformin, and methotrexate

d) bone marrow toxicity (aplastic anaemia) from drugs such as chloramphenicol, phenylbutazone and felbamate.

1.56   A E

Drugs produce their actions by acting upon receptors, ion channels and enzymes. Most receptors are present on the plasma membrane, although oestrogen and steroid receptors are located within the cytosol and nucleus. Receptors interacting with G proteins can either modulate adenylate cyclase activity or activate phospholipase C. Insulin acts on cells by interacting with a receptor which has an extracellular hormone-binding domain and a cytoplasmic enzyme domain with protein tyrosine kinase activity. When tissues are continuously exposed to an agonist, the numbers of receptors decrease or there is receptor desensitisation; this may cause tachyphylaxis (loss of efficacy with repeated doses).

1.57   A C E

Patients with peptic ulcer who are infected with *Helicobacter pylori* have been shown to benefit from eradication therapy. However, there is little evidence that patients with non-specific dyspepsia will benefit from treatment with antibiotics. The use of antisecretory drugs in   *H. pylori* infected patients reverses the predominantly antral pattern of gastritis and increases the severity of corpus gastritis. The pattern of gastritis then resembles that more commonly associated with the development of mucosal atrophy. There is accumulating epidemiological evidence suggesting an association between *H. pylori* infection and cancer of the gastric corpus and antrum. Eradication therapy, of which there are numerous regimens, generally has a success rate in excess of 90%.

1.58   B C

Patients who are HCV-RNA positive with chronic hepatitis on biopsy should be considered for treatment with α-interferon. Normalisation of serum transaminases is seen in 50% of patients, but in half of these, transaminase levels rise again after stopping therapy. The sustained response rate is 15–25%; those individuals most likely to develop severe liver disease may be the least likely to respond to antiviral treatment. Treatment is contraindicated in patients with autoimmune disease, active psychiatric disorder, alcohol abuse, decompensated liver disease and pregnancy. Fever, headache and myalgia (which can be alleviated by pre-treatment with paracetamol), anorexia and fatigue are common side-effects, while bone marrow suppression, alopecia, seizures, retinopathy and psychosis are rarer adverse effects.

1.59   B D E

Angiotensin-II receptor antagonists such as losartan (like ACE inhibitors) can be used in the treatment of hypertension and heart failure. Preliminary evidence suggests that they are as effective as ACE inhibitors in these conditions. Angiotensin-II receptor antagonists however do not block the degradation of bradykinin and therefore are less likely to cause cough and angioedema. Like ACE inhibitors, they are contraindicated in pregnancy and in patients with bilateral renal artery stenosis.

1.60   C E

Benzylpenicillin should be administered immediately in patients with suspected meningococcal disease. Studies investigating the utility of steroids have largely been performed in patients with meningitis caused by either *H. influenzae* or *Pneumococcus*; steroids have generally reduced the frequency of adverse neurological outcomes including deafness. However, the use of steroids has not been adequately studied in patients with meningococcal meningitis and the routine use, particularly in septicaemia, cannot be recommended at present. Chemoprophylaxis with rifampicin or ciprofloxacin is indicated for household or intimate contacts, but not for health-care workers unless they have given mouth-to-mouth resuscitation or inhaled respiratory secretions. Third generation cephalosporins are the mainstay of treatment in all forms of bacterial meningitis in all age groups. Cefuroxime however has been shown to be inferior to ceftriaxone and should not be used.

1.61   A B C E

Tinnitus and deafness are seen in salicylate poisoning of any severity. Salicylates directly stimulate the respiratory centre to increase the depth and rate of respiration, causing a respiratory alkalosis. A variable degree of metabolic acidosis is also present because of the loss of bicarbonate. Increased tissue glycolysis and increased peripheral demand for glucose can cause hypoglycaemia. Salicylates have a warfarin-like action on the vitamin K_1-epoxide cycle and can lead to hypoprothrombinaemia. Peptic ulceration is a feature of chronic salicylate therapy and not of acute poisoning.

1.62   D E

Neuroleptic malignant syndrome is an idiosyncratic reaction to therapeutic doses of phenothiazines, thioxanthines and butyro-phenones. It develops insidiously over 1–3 days, and is characterised by hyperthermia, muscle rigidity, impaired consciousness and tachycardia, and elevated creatine phosphokinase levels. Dantrolene but not calcium channel blockers may be of value. The mechanism responsible for the condition is unknown.

1.63   B C D E

Adenosine is of little use in atrial fibrillation. Digoxin toxicity can lead to most types of arrhythmias including atrial fibrillation. Sotalol has both class II and class III antiarrhythmic properties, and can be used in both ventricular and supraventricular tachycardias. Propafenone is a class Ic drug with actions on sodium channels, calcium channels and β-blocking activity. Prolonged Q-T interval may lead to torsades des pointes, which is difficult to treat with other antiarrhythmics, but may respond to magnesium.

1.64   A C

Zidovudine and acyclovir are often used together in patients with AIDS without any harmful effects. Aspirin and streptokinase were shown in ISIS-2 to have a beneficial effect in patients with acute myocardial infarction. Naproxen and penicillamine are often used together in patients with rheumatoid arthritis. Rifabutin metabolism can be inhibited by clarithromycin which may result in anterior uveitis. Sildenafil use is contraindicated in patients on nitrates since this can lead to dangerous hypotension.

1.65   B

The spontaneous adverse drug reaction (ADR) reporting scheme in the UK is termed the yellow card scheme. Reporting is voluntary; it is recommended that all serious ADRs and *all* ADRs to new drugs (marked by ▼ in the BNF) should be reported. Doctors, dentists, coroners and more recently pharmacists are allowed to report on yellow cards. It has been estimated that only 10% of all serious ADRs and 3–4% of all ADRs are actually reported; such gross under-reporting means that the yellow card data cannot be used to estimate the frequency of a particular ADR. Yellow card reports provide a signal that a drug may have the propensity to cause a particular ADR; this can provide the impetus for further epidemiological studies to allow a causal relationship to be established between an ADR and a drug.

1.66   B C E

Distribution volume is the volume of fluid in which the drug appears to distribute with a concentration equal to that in plasma. It can be calculated from a knowledge of the dose and concentration as long as the drug has linear kinetics. Thus, for a drug that remains within the circulation, the distribution volume will be similar to the blood volume, i.e. 5 litres. The distribution volume can be significantly higher than that of body water if the drug is distributed mainly within peripheral tissues. For example, the volume of distribution of chloroquine is 13,000l. Those drugs with a low Vd are mainly within the plasma and thus can be removed by haemodialysis, particularly in overdose situations.

1.67   A B E

The tryptophan loading test can be used to assess vitamin B_6 status, except in patients receiving oestrogens or with increased secretion of corticosteroids. Vitamin B_6 deficiency can be induced by penicillamine, and isoniazid (which increases urinary excretion). Cycloserine and hydralazine are antagonists of vitamin B_6. The liver plays a major role in the metabolism of pyridoxine. Pyridoxine can be used in pregnant women, for example in patients with hyperemesis gravidarum. Pyridoxine should not be given to patients receiving L-dopa as the action of L-dopa is antagonised. However, the vitamin can be used if the preparation contains both L-dopa and the dopa decarboxylase inhibitor carbidopa. High doses of pyridoxine may lead to sensory nerve damage and be manifested as paraesthesiae; this is reversible on stopping vitamin B_6.

1.68   A D

The mainstay of treatment for thyrotoxicosis are the thionamides (carbimazole and propylthiouracil). Both inhibit the iodination of tyrosine and coupling of iodotyrosines. In addition, propylthiouracil inhibits the peripheral conversion of T_4 to T_3. It usually takes 4–8 weeks for these drugs to have an effect. In that time, β-blockers are useful: they block the adrenergic effects of excess thyroid hormone such as sweating and tremor, but have no effect on basal metabolic rate. In euthyroid subjects, an excess of iodide from any source can cause a goitre. Radioactive iodine emits mainly β radiation (90%) which penetrates only 0.5 mm of tissue. It does emit some of the more penetrating γ rays which can be detected with a Geiger counter.

1.69   A C E

Methanol is eliminated in humans by oxidation to formaldehyde, formic acid and carbon dioxide. This is catalysed by the enzyme alcohol dehydrogenase. Blurred vision with a clear sensorium occurs 8–36 hours after poisoning, although optic atrophy is a late finding. Blood methanol levels should be determined as soon as possible. Methanol levels in excess of 50 mg/dl are thought to be an absolute indication for haemodialysis and ethanol treatment. The latter inhibits methanol oxidation by competing for alcohol dehydrogenase. Patients with methanol poisoning usually have a metabolic acidosis with an elevated anion gap.

1.70   A B C D

Drugs that inhibit the oxidation of acetaldehyde can cause a systemic reaction if taken with alcohol. This is the basis for the use of disulfiram as aversive treatment for alcoholism. Metronidazole can also inhibit acetaldehyde oxidation. Tinidazole may also have the same effect. Other drugs that can lead to flushing with alcohol include procarbazine, chlorpropamide, ketoconazole and cephamandole. Naltrexone is used in the treatment of alcoholics.

1.71   A D

Resistance to antibiotics is increasing largely because of the indiscriminate, widespread and inappropriate use of antibiotics. In general, resistance to penicillins is seen in more than 20% of isolates of methicillin-resistant *Staphylococcus aureus* (MRSA), *E. coli*, *Enterobacter* and *Acinetobacter*. Resistance is unknown in β-haemolytic streptococci and *N. meningitidis*. Less than 20% of isolates of *Pseudomonas*, *N. gonorrhoea*, *H. influenzae* and *Strep. pneumoniae* are resistant to penicillins.

1.72   A B E

Low molecular weight heparins (LMWHs) have mean molecular weights in the range 4–6 kDa. Compared with unfractionated heparin (UFH), they are weaker inhibitors of thrombin (factor IIa), but inhibit the coagulation enzyme Xa to a similar extent. Elimination of LMWHs is mainly via the kidneys, and is therefore likely to be reduced in patients with renal failure. Current evidence suggests that the risk of bleeding is similar with both sets of compounds. Immune mediated thrombocytopenia occurs with both LMWH and UFH; the risk may be lower with LMWH although this needs to be confirmed in larger studies. The osteopenic effect of LMWH may be less than that of UFH.

1.73   A B

In postmenopausal women, peripheral tissues are the main site of oestrogen production, usually by conversion of androstenedione and testosterone by aromatase to oestrone and oestradiol. These extra-glandular sites of oestrogen production can be inhibited by aromatase inhibitors. Aminoglutethimide was the first of these inhibitors but was rather non-specific causing inhibition of adrenal cortical enzymes as well. This necessitated the use of corticosteroid replacement. Anastrazole is a new generation aromatase inhibitor which is more potent and highly selective and thus does not affect adrenal function.

1.74   A B

Various drugs have been used for the treatment of obesity with varying degrees of success. Appetite suppressants such as fenfluramine and phentermine have been associated with primary pulmonary hypertension, and more recently with valvular heart disease. Although the prevalence of aortic and mitral regurgitation has varied in different studies, there is a consensus that these appetite suppressants lead to valvular heart disease (regurgitation rather than stenosis). The mechanism is unknown but may be related to increased production of serotonin (akin to the valve lesions seen in carcinoid syndrome). There is no evidence at the time of publication of this book that SSRIs (which are used for treatment of obesity) also lead to valvular heart disease.

1.75   A C E

Priapism is a prolonged and painful erection that cannot be relieved by sexual fulfilment. It has been reported in association with:

* phenothiazines, including chlorpromazine, promazine and fluphenazine
* the butyrophenone haloperidol
* trazodone but not conventional tricyclic antidepressants
* alpha-adrenoceptor antagonists including prazosin, phenoxybenzamine and labetalol
* warfarin
* intracavernosal papaverine

1.76   B C E

Sodium valproate is a broad-spectrum anticonvulsant. It has been used in patients with generalised seizures including myoclonic epilepsy, and partial seizures. Sodium valproate is teratogenic causing a valproate embryopathy syndrome and neural tube defects. It causes weight gain probably due to hypothalamic stimulation. Severe liver toxicity is a feared adverse effect which is more common in children, particularly those children with mental handicap on multiple enzyme-inducing anticonvulsants. Pancreatitis has also been reported with rechallenge causing recurrence of the pancreatitis.

IMMUNOLOGY: 'BEST OF FIVE' ANSWERS

2.1   D: Interleukin-2 (IL-2) and interferon-gamma (IFNγ)

T cells are classed on the basis of CD4 or CD8 surface-antigen expression, and on the production of cytokines. In the mouse two types of T-helper cells, TH1 and TH2, are associated with cell-mediated and humoral-mediated immunity respectively. The TH1 cells secrete interleukin-2 (IL-2) and interferon-gamma, and TH2 cells IL-4 and IL-10. Most human T-cells have both TH1 and TH2 activity.

Interleukins-2 and -15 induce T cell proliferation and IL-4 and -13 (both also secreted by T cells) encourage B-cell activation and proliferation. T cells also produce the endothelial activator TNFβ.

Macropahges secrete tumour necrosis factor alpha, IL-1, and IL-8. They also produce IL-10 (as do T cells), and IL-12 (as do B cells). Tumour necrosis factor alpha regulates cell growth and stimulates leucocytes and adhesion receptor induction.

Transforming growth factor beta (TGFβ) is a product of T cells and monocytes. It promotes humoral immunity, reducing the acute inflammatory reaction and inhibiting cell growth.

Interferon alpha and beta are produced principally by leucocytes and fibroblasts respectively, and induce adaptations in unaffected cells that increase protection against viral invasion.

2.2   B: B-cell/bone marrow

Immune surveillance or 'tolerance' is an important process that reduces auto-reactivity to 'self'. Both primary (central) and secondary (peripheral) processes prevent auto-reactivity. For B-cells this occurs initially in the bone marrow and then peripherally in the spleen and lymph nodes. A peripheral mechanism is required because B-cells can continue to change and possibly express new immunoglobulins that are reactive to 'self'. The T-cell receptor does not undergo similar changes peripherally and therefore has only a central site of regulation that is in the thymus.

2.3   B: Di George syndrome

Primary immunodeficiency disorders tend to occur in childhood and are most often X-linked. Examples A, C and E above are B-cell defects. Wiskott-Aldrich syndrome (often manifest as thrombocytopenia and lymphopenia) and severe combined immunodeficieny have B-cell and T-cell defects. Ataxia telangiectasia is another condition associated with several deficiencies of immunoglobulins and lymphopenia. The Di George syndrome is a T-cell disorder, as are purine nucleoside phosphorylase deficiency and Bloom's syndrome. Other primary deficiencies of immunoregulation include complement receptor 3 deficiencies and the phagocyte disorders myeloperoxidase deficiency, Job's syndrome, and Chediak-Higashi syndrome.

Secondary immunodeficiency is much more common than primary disease and causes include therapies (chemotherapeutic drugs, corticosteroids, irradiation, plasmapheresis), viral infections (HIV, influenza), malignancies (solid tumours, lymphoproliferative disorders), autoimmune immune rheumatic diseases (systemic lupus erythematosus, dermatomyositis, vasculitis, rheumatoid arthritis), diabetes mellitus and poor nutrition.

2.4   A: Hepatitis C

Cryoglobulins are immunoglobulins that precipitate at a temperature of 40°C. There are three categories of cryoglobulin, Type I monoclonal immunoglobulin, Type II mixed monoclonal/polyclonal, and Type III polyclonal immunoglobulin. Type I disorders include examples B and E. Type III disorders include examples C and D. Hepatitis C, Sjögren's syndrome, and lymphoproliferative disorders are associated with Type II cryoglobulinaemia.

Common clinical manifestations of cryoglobulinaemia include arthralgia, cutaneous vasculitis, hepatitis, and muscle weakness (rarely myositis). Rarer complaints include Raynaud's phenomenon, hyperviscosity syndrome, and neuropathies.

2.5   A: The Fab portion of one heavy chain linked to one light chain

A Fab fragment is monovalent and is generated by papain digestion of immunoglobulin. The Fab fragment is made up of an intact light chain and the N-terminal variable heavy and constant H1 domains of the heavy chain.

IMMUNOLOGY: MULTIPLE CHOICE ANSWERS

2.6   A C E

Via the alternative pathway, Bb (cleaved from factor B by factor D) binds to C3b to form the unstable C3bBb (equivalent to C3 convertase of the classical pathway). The compound is then stabalised by properidin. C3-nephritic factor (found in some cases of membrano-proliferative GN type II) is an autoantibody that stabilises C3bBb; the positive feedback amplification of the alternative pathway cascade then consumes C3 (but not C4). Factor H can bind to C3b and, by acting as a cofactor, allows factor I to inactive C3b, controlling further activation of the pathway. The classical pathway is activated by antigen–antibody complexes binding to multiple domain C1q; the pentameric head of IgM makes this the most efficient stimulant.

2.7   A C

Secretory IgA is dimeric, the two subunits joined by a J-chain; IgM is pentameric. IgA and IgE can fix complement via the alternative pathway; IgG and IgM via the classical pathway. Of the normal total immunoglobulin pool IgG makes up approx 75%, IgA 15% and IgM 10%. There are traces of IgD and IgE. Only IgG can cross the placenta. The constant region of the molecule (Fc) determines the class of immunoglobulin. The Fab region has a variable (V) and constant (CH) domain, the former being unique for each antibody.

2.8   A C D

Certain HLA alleles are associated with increased risk of disease. The following are further examples: A3/B14 in haemochromatosis; A28 in schizophrenia; B5 in Behçet's disease and ulcerative colitis; DR3/7 DQW2 in coeliac disease; B27 in ankylosing spondylitis and psoriatic arthropathy; DR2 in Goodpasture's syndrome and narcolepsy; DR3 in chronic active hepatitis, Grave's disease, myasthenia gravis, Addison's disease and Sjögren's syndrome; DR4 in rheumatoid arthritis and insulin dependent diabetes, and DR5 in Hashimoto's thyroiditis.

2.9   B

Esterified fatty acids are converted to arachidonic acid via phospholipase A2; this reaction is inhibited by corticosteroids. Arachidonic acid is then converted to leukotrienes via 5-lipoxygenase, and prostaglandins via cyclo-oxygenase. NSAIDs block prostaglandin synthesis. Two subtypes of COX have been identified. COX 1 activation leads to the production of prostacyclin, is antithrombogenic and cytoprotective in the gastric mucosa. It is now thought that the inhibition of inflammation by NSAIDs is mostly a consequence of inhibiting COX2 and that the inhibition of COX1 leads to gastric side-effects; thus NSAID with high COX2 to COX1 activity ratio (selective COX2 inhibition) may have good anti-inflammatory action with fewer side-effects.

2.10   B D E

Complement activation by the 'alternative pathway' occurs in the absence of antibodies by hydrolysis of C3 to C3b by substances such as endotoxin. Increased capillary permeability is largely due to the release of histamine from mast cells in response to C3a and C5a. These factors are also chemotactic for neutrophils. Lysis of cells coated with complement is a function of the late complement components C8 and C9, which create holes in cell membranes. Heat treatment is the standard laboratory method for inactivating complement.

INFECTIOUS DISEASES: 'BEST OF FIVE'
ANSWERS

3.1   A: Acute HBV infection

Hepatitis B surface antigen (HBsAg) is an early indicator of acute infection. If it persists for more than 6 months in the presence of IgG antibodies to the core (anti-HBc IgG) it would suggest a chronic carrier state. Antibodies to HbsAg indicate recovery and immunity and are found after successful immunization.

Anti-HBc IgM appear early in infection and persist during acute infection. The IgG subclass persists for life and indicates previous exposure to the hepatitis B virus.

The 'e' antigen is associated with infectivity and is usually present for 3–6 weeks, rising and falling within the time span of a raised HbsAg. A persistent 'e' antigen would suggest a chronic carrier status.

3.2   E: Rotavirus

The options are all examples of human RNA viruses. Rotavirus infection occurs mainly in childhood and is associated with respiratory symptoms and diarrhoea. Arboviruses include yellow fever and dengue; arena viruses, Lassa fever and epidemic haemorrhagic fever. Picornavirus is associated with haemorrhagic conjunctivitis and an atypical form of measles, a paramyxovirus, is associated with severe illness and haemorrhage.

3.3   D: Melarsoprol is effective treatment

African trypanosomiasis follows the bite of the tsetse fly and the transfer of *T. brucei*. Humans are an important reservoir for the protozoan. The Rhodesian and Gambian forms of the disease are similar clinically except that Rhodesian sleeping sickness tends to be acute and severe rather than chronic and indolent, and death from Rhodesian disease often occurs within one year. Fever, lymphadenopathy, hepatosplenomegaly, and CNS disease are common features. Suramin and pentamidine are useful therapies but do not cross the blood-brain barrier. CNS disease is best treated with melarsoprol but it is not effective in Rhodesian sleeping sickness.

3.4   B: *P. falciparum*

In humans, the malaria life cycle starts with the injection of the infective sporozoite through the skin by the Anopheles mosquito. During pre-erythrocytic schizogony sporozoites mature to micromerozoites in the liver and are then liberated into the bloodstream and infect red blood cells. It is in the ensuing erythrocytic stage that micromerozoites transform through a trophozoite and shizont phase to become the 'asexual' merozoites that are typically seen on a blood film. Some of these merozoites develop into 'sexual' gametocytes and at this stage the patient becomes infective.

A fourth exoerythrocytic phase exists. This occurs in the liver. A variable number of original sporozoites remain latent in the liver, not transforming to micromerozoites. In this way there appears to be a cycle of continuous re-infection. This phenomenon is definitely seen with *P. vivax*, probably occurs with *P. ovale*, and possibly occurs with *P. malariae*. It is not a feature of the life cycle of *P. falciparum*. It is for this reason that primaquine is required for the eradication of *P. vivax, P. ovale,* and *P. malariae*, as it has an effect on the exoerythrocytic cycle.

3.5   A: Cysticercosis

Cysticercosis occurs after ingesting the eggs of *Taenia solium* (pork tapeworm). It is seen in areas of Asia, Africa and South America. Cysterci may develop in any tissue of the body but are most commonly found as space-occupying cerebral lesions and subcutaneous nodules. Retinitis, uveitis, conjunctivitis, choroidal atrophy and blindness may also occur. The treatment of choice is praziquantel.

3.6   D: The Weil-Felix reaction is positive

Q fever is caused by the rickettsia-like organism *Coxiella burnetii*. Although the Weil-Felix agglutination test is being replaced by a complement-fixation test, it is still useful. The test relies on the presence of a common antigen found on some *Rickettsia* and on *Proteus*. It is positive in the typhus fevers but negative in rickettsial pox, trench fever, and Q fever.

Coxiella burnetii is widespread in domestic and farm animals and is spread by a host tick. Modes of spread to man are thought to include cows' milk, aerosol and dust.

There is usually a fever with a 'flu-like illness that may resolve or progress to pneumonia or endocarditis. Epididymo-orchitis, uveitis and osteomyelitis have also been documented. Tetracycline is the treatment of choice.

3.7   B: All of the options

Any impairment of host immunity, including chronic alcohol abuse, may add to the risk of an atypical infection. Healthy adults are usually immune having developed capsular and specific bacterial related antibodies, either directly related to *Haemophilus* exposure or through cross-reactivity with other common Gram-negative bacteria.

3.8   D: Leptospirosis

Infectious mononucleosis should be considered but the clinical features and risk associated with occupation point towards the spirochaetal infection, leptospirosis

(Weil's disease). The early, leptospiraemic phase is characterised by constitutional symptoms of fever, malaise, weight loss, and headache. Infrequently there may be a rash, lymphadenopathy, or hepatosplenomegaly. During the second phase of the infection 50% of cases complain of meningism. Most cases will resolve spontaneously but a small number develop renal impairment, haematuria, haemolytic anaemia, jaundice and cardiac failure.

The organism can be cultured from blood or cerebrospinal fluid in the first week. Serological tests for IgM antibodies are useful. Penicillin or erythromycin are suitable treatments.

3.9   D: None of the options

Epidermolytic toxins of S. *aureus* cause scalded skin syndrome. This is indistinguishable from toxic epidermal necrolysis which has a number of additional causes. However, given the number of staphylococcal infections, the association is uncommon. Toxic shock syndrome is mediated by toxins TSST1 and enterotoxins B and C; bacteraemia is rare and treatment is mainly supportive though antibiotics are required to eradicate the focal source. A rapid onset of septicaemia is an infrequent complication of streptococcal cellulitis. Group A beta-haemolytic *Strep. pyogenes* is associated with erysipelas in the elderly. Impetigo is usually superficial not affecting the dermis. Ecthyma is an ulcerating form of impetigo extending into the dermis. Both forms are associated with increased risk of glomerulonephritis.

3.10   A: All of the options

Atypical infections might also include *Nocardia*, *Candida*, *Mycoplasma*, *Mycobacterium*, cytomegalovirus, *Aspergillus*, and *Pneumocystis*.

3.11   D: *Staphylococcus aureus* endocarditis and septicaemia

This is a description of *Staphylococcus aureus* septicaemia, tricuspid endocarditis and septic pulmonary emboli in an intravenous drug user. Confusion is common in severe sepsis and does not always indicate intracranial infection, although this must always be considered. *Streptococcus bovis* endocarditis would typically be less acute, and is associated with underlying gastrointestinal disease (especially bowel cancer) rather than intravenous drug use.

3.12   C: Clarithromycin

Macrolides such as erythromycin and clarithromycin interfere with bacterial ribosomal function. The β-lactam agents, such as amoxycillin, and glycopeptides, such as vancomycin, act by inhibiting cell wall synthesis. The fluoroquinolone ciprofloxacin inhibits bacterial DNA supercoiling by acting on DNA gyrase and topoisomerase enzymes. Trimethoprim is a diaminopyrimidine that acts by inhibiting folic acid synthesis.

3.13   A: *Listeria monocytogenes*

Neonates, the elderly and immunocompromised individuals are at increased risk of *Listeria* meningitis. Pregnant women are prone to listerial bacteraemia, but meningitis is rare; the baby rather than the mother is at risk of central nervous system infection. Amoxycillin or benzylpenicillin are the treatments of choice in listerial meningitis. Cephalosporins are not effective. The CSF findings in listerial meningitis are often only mildly abnormal. The glucose level may be normal, a lymphocytic picture may predominate, and the Gram-stain is often negative; a partially treated meningitis of any cause could have similar CSF findings.

3.14   C: Nephritis

CMV infection in HIV positive individuals (and other immunocompromised patients) is associated with a large variety of presentations. Important manifestations include CNS infection (retinitis, encephalitis, polyradiculopathy, myelitis), gastro-intestinal disease (oesophagitis, colitis, acalculous cholecystitis, hepatitis) and pulmonary involvement (interstitial pneumonitis – much less of a problem in HIV infection than in post-transplant patients). Although urinary shedding of CMV occurs in viraemic patients, CMV nephritis has not been recognised as a significant complication of infection.

3.15   A: CCR5

The *Gp120*, gag gene product, and protease enzyme are all viral products rather than host-derived. CD8+ is not involved in HIV attachment. CCR5 is now recognised to be a crucial co-receptor in the HIV replication cycle. Mutations of the gene that codes for this co-receptor have been shown to be protective against HIV infection.

3.16   E: Schistosomiasis

Schistosomiasis usually presents as a chronic disease, typically with liver (principally *Schistosoma mansoni*, *S. japonicum*), bowel (*S. mansoni*, *S. japonicum*) or urinary tract (*S. haematobium*) involvement. However, acute schistosomiasis ('Katayama fever') may also occur. The clinical picture in acute schistosomiasis is dominated by allergic phenomena including fever, urticaria, marked eosinophilia, diarrhoea, hepatosplenomegaly and wheeze.

Amoebiasis and visceral leishmaniasis might explain the diarrhoea and hepatosplenomegaly respectively, but not the wheeze, urticaria and eosinophilia.

3.17   B: JC virus

This is a clinical picture suggestive of the demyelinating disease progressive multifocal leukoencephalopathy (PML) caused by the JC virus. It typically presents over a period of weeks with focal weakness, slurring of speech, gait disturbance and changes in mental state. Patients are generally afebrile, and CSF analysis is usually normal though polymerase chain reaction (PCR) assays for JC virus may be positive. Imaging with MRI reveals focal or diffuse white-matter lesions that do not enhance with contrast or display mass effect.

The other pathogens above can cause CNS infection, but none fits the overall clinical scenario as well as JC virus. *Cryptococcus neoformans* and *Mycobacterium tuberculosis* would typically cause a sub-acute meningitis (with CSF abnormalities), whilst single or multiple ring-enhancing lesions are seen in cerebral toxoplasmosis. *Nocardia asteroides* is a rare cause of brain abscess in the immunocompromised.

3.18   D: Toxic Shock Syndrome

Not every patient who presents with vomiting and diarrhoea has got gastro-enteritis! The clinical picture here is a classic one for staphylococcal toxic shock syndrome (TSS). The criteria required for a diagnosis of TSS are:

Temperature ≥ 38.5°C

Hypotension (systolic BP < 90 mmHg)

Rash with subsequent desquamation, particularly on palms and soles

Involvement of at least 3 of the following organ/systems:

GI (diarrhoea, vomiting)

Musculoskeletal (severe myalgia or raised CPK)

Mucous membranes (hyperaemia of conjunctivae, pharynx or vagina)

Renal (renal impairment)

Hepatic (abnormal LFTs)

Thrombocytopenia

CNS (disorientation without focal neurology).

Other conditions must also be excluded (e.g. measles).

3.19   C: Genital herpes

The description is typical of genital herpes, probably HSV-2. His country of origin is irrelevant in this case. If he entered the UK recently then 'exotic' STDs such as chancroid and LGV would need to be considered, but the clinical presentation is not suggestive of either of these. Syphilis (painless, smooth ulcers) must always be considered in genital ulcer disease, but again the clinical picture does not fit with this or with Behçet's disease.

3.20   E: Toxic side-effects of isoniazid are best reduced by the concomitant use of rifabutin

Rifampicin, isoniazid, ethambutol, rifabutin, and pyrazinamide are commonly used anti-tuberculous drugs. Rifampicin and isoniazid may cause hepatitis. The toxic effects of isoniazid also include peripheral neuritis and lupus-like symptoms, and can be reduced by the concomitant use of pyrazinamide. Rifabutin causes uveitis, the risk of this is raised by the concomitant use of macrolide antibiotics or triazole antifungals; the dose of rifabutin should be reduced in this situation. Capreomycin is reserved for drug-resistant cases and is associated with nephrotoxicity, ototoxicity, hepatitis and eosinophilia.

INFECTIOUS DISEASES: MULTIPLE CHOICE ANSWERS

3.21   B C E

Membrane glycoproteins gp41 and gp120 are encoded on the 'env' gene and gp120 specifically binds to the CD4 receptor. The transmembrane protein gp41 is involved in the fusion of viral envelope and host cell membrane. The HIV genome is a diploid of two single-stranded RNA. A DNA provirus is inserted into the host DNA. The virus can cause direct renal toxicity. Renal drug induced toxicity is seen with amphotericin B, foscarnet and co-trimoxazole. Polyclonal activation of B cells tends to increase immunoglobulin secretion.

3.22   B C D

Prions are defined as 'proteinaceous infectious particles that resist inactivation by procedures which modify nucleic acids'. The normal protein PrPc is protease sensitive and no different to PrPsc in amino acid sequence. Post-translational processes modify PrPc to the infectious PrPsc. Some families with inherited prion disease have a late onset and lower risk of symptoms if heterozygous at codon 129 for methionine and valine as opposed to homozygous for either amino acid. Other amino acid substitutions are also documented both as point mutations and insertions. Biopsy is the only absolute diagnostic test in Creutzfeldt–Jakob disease. The EEG may show a characteristic 'pseudo periodic' wave activity.

3.23   D

Except for pneumococcal vaccine which is a polysaccharide, the above false answers are all 'inactivated'. Other 'inactivated' vaccines include typhus, plague and Q fever. The BCG, measles, mumps, rubella and yellow fever vaccines are 'live-attenuated'. One of three available vaccines for typhoid is live-attenuated. At the time of writing the old rabies vaccine is live-attenuated but not the new and there are trials underway on a live attenuated vaccine for cholera.

3.24   A B C D E

A complete list of notifiable diseases can be obtained from your microbiology department; the following examples are notifiable: anthrax, cholera, diphtheria, Haemophilus Influenzae B meningitis, hepatitis A and B, measles, mumps, rubella, menningococcal and pneumococcal meningitis, pertussis, poliomyelitis, rabies, smallpox, tetanus, tuberculosis, typhoid and Yellow fever. Varicella (chickenpox) is notifiable in Scotland and Northern Ireland.

3.25   A B C D

In the normal life cycle *S.mansoni* and *S.japonicum* migrate to the mesenteric and portal veins and *S.haematobium* to the pelvic veins and vesical plexus; the first two shed eggs into the intestine and *S.haematobium* into the bladder. Ectopic ova may be found in the CNS. Praziquantel is the treatment of choice. *S.mansoni* also responds to oxamniquine and *S.haematobium* to metriphonate, however these treatments are virtually obsolete. In the presence of porto-caval shunting, *S.mansoni* and *S.japonicum* are deposited in the pulmonary vessels, leading to fibrosis and arteritis, in turn causing pulmonary hypertension. Recurrent infection in endemic areas is common. Any required immunity is, on the whole, inefficient.

3.26   A E

The onset of disease is usually non-specific. Neurological signs may be absent but in severe disease confusion, ataxia, focal symptoms and seizures may occur. Jaundice is a feature in less than 10% of cases. Hepatic failure is not a recognised complication. Some rickettsial illnesses, such as scrub typhus and tick typhus have an eschar at the site of infection, whereas others such as Rocky Mountain spotted fever and epidemic typhus are not associated with eschar formation. Serological markers are of little use in the first week of illness. Oral deoxycycline is the treatment of choice but chloramphenicol can be given intravenously and during pregnancy.

3.27   D

The most common cause (40–50%) of non-specific (non-gonococcal) urethritis is *Chlamydia trachomatis* (type D and E). Approximately 25% of cases have no known cause. *Chlamydia* infection is best treated with tetracycline. Epididymitis and urethral strictures are uncommon. *C. trachomatis* is also commonly responsible for PID. Other organisms to consider include *Mycoplasma hominis* and *M. genitalium* and *Actinomyces israelli* (often associated with plastic intra-uterine devices).

3.28   B C E

Insect bites are responsible for the spread of yellow fever, malaria and dengue (mosquito), African trypanosomiasis (tse-tse fly), onchocerciasis (black fly), Leishmaniasis (sandfly), Chagas disease (reduviid bug) and tick borne *Borreliosis* and tularaemia. Contact with an infected person can lead to direct infection with Marburg and Ebola virus. Lassa fever is spread by contamination with rat urine and faeces as is hantavirus (Korean heamorrhagic fever).

3.29   D

Visceral and cutaneous leishmaniasis can be treated with pentavalent antimony compounds. Trypanosomiasis is treated with suramin, pentamidine, melarsoprol (Gambian type) and nitrofurazone (CNS disease and Chagas' disease). Several clinical forms of toxoplasmosis occur ranging from asymptomatic lymphadenopathy, through an infectious mononucleosis like (Paul Bunnell negative) state to an acute febrile illness with maculopapular rash, organomegaly, uveitis, hepatitis and myocarditis. *Entamoeba histolytica* causes amoebiasis. *Giardia* can be excreted intermittently. Duodenal aspirate and jejunal biopsy may demonstrate the parasite.

3.30   A E

Hepatitis A faecal shedding occurs late in incubation and in the prodromal phase. Contacts should receive pooled globulin or active immunisation. Treatment of acute hepatitis is supportive; steroids are not indicated though pulsed steroids along with alpha interferon may be of benefit in chronic hepatitis B and C. The Hbs Ag antigen is present in acute and chronic hepatitis B; high titres of IgM anti HBC (core) indicates acute infection or seroconversion illness in a chronic eAg positive patient. Hepatitis E, like A, does not progress to chronic disease and is not associated with increased risk of carcinoma. Recovery is seen in 30% of hepatitis C patients. Of the remainder, 60% persist with chronic hepatitis and up to 10% may go on to develop cirrhosis and/or hepatic carcinoma.

3.31   A B

Mycoplasma do not have a cell wall and do not Gram stain. Pontiac fever is a short lived flu-like illness caused by legionella. It is not associated with pneumonia. It is thought to be due to inhalation of antigen from dead bacteria. Whilst serology is useful in the diagnosis of legionella (titres peaking at 4–8 weeks), they are not specific and cross react with other organisms, including E.coli and campylobacter.

3.32   B E

Brucella is a Gram-negative non-spore-forming intracellular aerobe. Typically it can be found in unpasteurized milk and soil for up to 8 weeks. The white cell count is usually normal but there may be a leucopenia and relative lymphocytosis. The UK is considered a disease free country; the incidence of the disease worldwide is increasing. Common modes of transmission are inhalation, ingestion of raw meat and untreated milk, and penetrating skin wounds. Transplacental and breast milk transfer may also occur.

3.33   A B E

Most infection with *C. immitis* is asymptomatic; occasionally pneumonia, arthralgia, erythema nodosum or multiforme, and meningism are reported. Most disease caused by *Aspergillus* is due to *A. fumigatus*. Paranasal granulomata are caused by *A. flavus,* and otomycosis by *A. niger.* Cryptococcal pneumonia is less common than meningitis. Blastomycosis is confirmed by culture or histology. There is cross reactivity with histoplasma antibodies.

3.34   B D

Isoniazid inhibits phenytoin and carbamazepine metabolism. Rifampicin is an hepatic enzyme inducer; rare side effects include thrombocytopenic purpura, haemolytic anaemia and acute renal failure. Pyrazinamide inhibits renal uric acid secretion. Ethambutol has ocular toxicity; streptomycin is ototoxic. The latter is also a weak neuromuscular blocker and causes a cutaneous hypersensitivity reaction. A transient, small enzyme rise is common with several of these agents. Hepatitis usually resolves rapidly on discontinuing therapy, but can be severe and fatal incidences have occured. Hepatotoxicity has been associated in the main with Pyrazinamide, Rifampicin and Isoniazid (in descending order of importance).

3.35   A C D

Cryptosporidia and *Microsporidia* account for 40% of infective diarrhoea; cytomegalovirus 20%, *M. avium intracellular* 10%, and *Giardia* 5%. *Pneumocystis carinii* pneumonia is not thought to arise by reactivation of latent infection but from airborne re-infection. Early in infection the chest radiograph may appear normal. Bilateral interstitial infiltrate is common but consolidation can occur. Tuberculosis can stimulate cell-mediated immunity there-by activating HIV production in infected T cells. Most CNS infection occurs late. Early, uncommon encephalopathies and presumed autoimmune disorders are reported. Classic infections include cryptococcal meningitis, cortical (grey matter) toxoplasmosis, and demyelination by JC virus (progressive multifocal leucoencephalopathy) and generally HIV encephalopathy is a late manifestation.

3.36   B C E

Radiotherapy and resection are the best treatments for focal Kaposi lesions; systemic disease can be treated with vincristine, bleomycin and anthracycline. Large cell lymphomas in the immunocompromised transplant patient are nearly always associated with EBV. This is true of 50% of AIDS associated lymphomas except in the CNS which, like the transplant case, are nearly always positive for EBV. Peripheral nerve and muscle infection is uncommon. Cytomegalovirus (CMV) can cause a painful, ascending polyradiculopathy and mononeuritis multiplex. Cotton wool spots are seen in 50% of patients and are usually visual sparing and non-infectious, requiring no treatment. They may be associated with increased risk of CMV retinitis and confused with the latter. AIDS related sclerosing cholangitis is caused by several agents including cryptosporidia, microsporidia and CMV.

3.37   D

Visceral and cutaneous leishmaniasis can be treated with pentavalent antimony compounds. Trypanosomiasis is treated with suramin, pentamidine, melarsoprol (Gambian type) and nitrofurazone (CNS disease and Chagas' disease). Several clinical forms of toxoplasmosis occur ranging from asymptomatic lymphadenopathy, through an infectious mononucleosis like (Paul Bunnell negative) state to an acute febrile illness with maculopapular rash, organomegaly, uveitis, hepatitis and myocarditis. *Entamoeba histolytica* causes amoebiasis. *Giardia* can be excreted intermittently. Duodenal aspirate and jejunal biopsy may demonstrate the parasite.

3.38   A B C D E

Other atypicals include *Mycoplasma, Mycobacterium,* cytomegalovirus, aspergillosis and pneumocystis.

3.39   B C

Pyrimidine and G6PD synthesis can occur *de novo*; purines are exogenous. *Plasmodium vivax* and *ovate,* but not *Plasmodium falciparum,* have a persisting hepatic cycle, from which late relapse can occur. The normal incubation period is 7–14 days, but this may be affected by concomitant antimalarial therapies. Regarding Falciparum malaria, 90% of patients present within one month and 99% within six months of leaving an endogenous area.

3.40   A B C D E

Lyme disease is characterised by erythema chronicum migrans, fever, arthralgia, myalgia, lymphadenopathy and neurological and cardiac complications. Louse-borne (epidemic) and tick-borne (endemic) relapsing fever are associated with hepatic and splenic tenderness and enlargement, jaundice, liver failure and DIC. Tetracycline treatment of louse and tick-borne disease can produce a sometimes fatal Jarisch–Herxheimer reaction. Steroids do not prevent the Jarisch–Herxheimer reaction in louse-borne relapsing fever unlike their effect in acute syphilis; they are however useful in helping to reduce temperature and hypotension. The reaction can also be reduced by meptazinol, an opiate antagonist, and polyclonal anti-tumour necrosis factor antibody.

RHEUMATOLOGY: 'BEST OF FIVE' ANSWERS

4.1   B: Any of these items

Non-steroidal anti-inflammatory drugs (NSAIDs) may interact with a number of different medications. Methotrexate and lithium levels may rise. Whilst a recognised interaction, it is very common to find patients on both methotrexate and an NSAID. Monitoring of the full blood count and liver function on a 4–6 week basis is essential with methotrexate treatment, whether taking NSAIDs or not.

The effectiveness of thiazides, loop diuretics, beta-blockers, ACE-inhibitors, and oral hypoglycaemic agents may fall. There is also an increased risk of hyperkaleamia with potassium-sparing diuretics.

The patient is also taking corticosteroids. This may increase the risk of gastro-intestinal bleeding and exacerbate fluid retention.

4.2   C: Use of a beta-blocker

Men over the age of 60-years may lose bone density, however, the risk of osteoporotic fracture does not appear to increase in males until after the age of 70. Other risk factors include hypogonadism (low testosterone levels), smoking, chronic alcohol abuse, lack of exercise, poor nutrition, drugs (such as corticosteroids, heparin, thyroxine, and phenytoin), and disorders such as rheumatoid arthritis, diabetes mellitus, chronic liver or renal disease, malabsorption syndromes, and endocrinopathies (Cushing's syndrome, hyperthyroidism, hyperparathyroidism). Low trauma fractures should be investigated with dual energy X-ray absorptiometry (DEXA) at all ages though there is an argument for commencing the elderly patient (> 80 years) on calcium and vitamin D without scanning, and/or newer bisphosphonates in the presence of new spinal fractures.

4.3   C: Drugs implicated to cause DIL should not be used in idiopathic systemic lupus erythematosus

Many drugs have been implicated in causing drug-induced lupus (DIL). Those definitely and most commonly associated with DIL are hydralazine, procainamide, isoniazid, quinidine, methyldopa, chlorpromazine, and salazopyrin. Hydralazine associated DIL is considered to be dose-dependent, and procainamide time-dependent. Up to 90% of cases taking procainamide develop a positive anti-nuclear antibody (ANA) and 30% of these develop DIL.

Renal, central nervous system and skin features of systemic lupus erythematosus (SLE) are rare in DIL. Other features of SLE such as articular, pulmonary and serosal disease are common.

In the majority of cases the condition subsides on withdrawing the drug. There is no contraindication to using these drugs in idiopathic SLE.

4.4   A: All of the following

The granular, diffuse and cytoplasm distributed c-ANCA affects the target antigen proteinase-3 and is associated with Wegener's granulomatosis. The peri-nuclear distributed p-ANCA binds to several enzymes including myeloperoxidase, and is associated with microscopic polyangiitis, polyarteritis nodosa, Churg-Strauss syndrome, Felty's syndrome and inflammatory bowel disease. An atypical peri-nuclear a-ANCA is found in inflammatory bowel diseases, endocarditis, and HIV.

4.5   A: A skin biopsy often demonstrates evidence of vasculitis

These features are consistent with familial Mediterranean fever (FMF), though the differential diagnosis might include, polyarteritis nodosa, porphyria, hereditary angio-oedema, rheumatic fever, or septic arthritis.

FMF is an autosomal recessive disorder. The genetic defect is on chromosome 16. Most cases (80%) present before the age of 20 years and most frequently in people of eastern Mediterranean descent (Armenians, Arabs and Sephardic and Ashkenazi Jews).

Serositis is common; 95% of cases have abdominal attacks and 50% pleural attacks. Arthritis occurs in 75% of cases and an erysipelas-like rash in up to 50% of cases. There may be erosive joint disease and the most common picture is a monoarthritis. This tends to resolve spontaneously over weeks to months. The skin lesions show a dermal infiltration of neutrophils rather than a vasculitis.

Amyloidosis can occur in up to 40% of cases leading to renal failure, proteinuria, or malabsorption. An elevated ESR, leucocytosis, normochromic normocytic anaemia, and inflammatory synovial fluid are all non-specific features. Colchicine may help. Corticosteroids are unhelpful.

4.6   D: Joint pains in more than one joint for one week

Hypermobility is considered present if a person satisfies four or more manoeuvres in the nine-point Beighton hypermobility score:

The ability to:	R	L
1. Passively dorsiflex the 5th metacarpo-phalangeal joint to ≥ 90°	1	1
2. Oppose the thumb to the volar aspect of the ipsilateral forearm	1	1
3. Hyperextend the elbow ≥ 10°	1	1
4. Hyperextend the knee ≥ 10°	1	1
5. Place hands flat on the floor without bending the knees		1
Total score	9	

Other joints, not included in this scoring system, may also be hypermobile and specialists in this area will take them into account when considering a diagnosis of hypermobility. Likewise, a history of being able to do these manoeuvres in the past is important when examining older patients whose levels of flexibility may now be reduced. Benign joint hypermobility syndrome (BJHS) is excluded in the presence of Marfan's or Ehlers-Danlos syndrome. The revised (Beighton 1988) criteria for BJHS are shown below. The BJHS is diagnosed in the presence of 2 major, 1 major and 2 minor, or 4 minor criteria. Two minor criteria will suffice where there is an unequivocally affected first-degree relative.

Major criteria:

1. A Beighton score of 4/9 or greater (either current or historical)
2. Arthralgia for longer than 3 months in 4 or more joints

Minor criteria:

1. A Beighton score of 1, 2 or 3/9
2. Arthralgia in 1–3 joints or back pain, either for longer than 3 months, spondylosis/spondylolisthesis
3. Dislocation/subluxation in more than one joint, or one joint on more than one occasion
4. Soft tissue rheumatism in 3 or more sites
5. Marfanoid habitus
6. Abnormal skin: straie, hyperextensibility, papyraceous scars
7. Eye signs: drooping eyelids, myopia, antimongoloid slant
8. Varicose veins, hernias, uterine/rectal prolapse

4.7   B: Serum uric acid levels are increased in Fanconi's syndrome

Increased levels of serum uric acid are seen in states of high purine turnover or reduced renal excretion. High purine turnover states include lympho- and myeloproliferative disorders, chemotherapy, psoriasis, haemolytic anaemia, and pregnancy. Reduced renal clearance may occur in renal failure, with use of diuretics (except spironolactone), low-dose salicylates, cyclosporin, ethambutol, pyrazinamide, alcohol, metabolic acidosis, hypothyroidism, hypo- and hyper-parathyroidism, and lead poisoning.

Uricosuric drugs reduce serum levels of uric acid. These include probenecid and high-dose salicylates. Fanconi's syndrome and Wilson's disease are both associated with decreased levels of serum uric acid.

Inherited metabolic syndromes of hyperuricaemia include Lesch-Nyhan syndrome (X-linked hypoxanthine guanine phosphoribosyl transferase deficiency) and von Gierke's disease (autosomal recessive glucose-6 phosphatase deficiency).

4.8 D: Systemic lupus erythematosus

Autoantibodies to dsDNA are found in up to 60% of cases of systemic lupus erythematosus (SLE). The antibody is associated with nephritis and severe disease. The autoantibody Sm is found in up to 40% of cases and associated with interstitial lung disease. It is very uncommon to find these autoantibodies in association with other autoimmune rheumatic diseases.

Autoantibodies to snRNP are also common in SLE, but are less specific and may be found in overlap syndromes with features of polymyositis and systemic sclerosis. Anti-Ro and anti-La antibodies may be found in 10–30% of SLE patients. They are, however, more commonly associated with Sjögren's syndrome.

Less than 5% of SLE cases will have the autoantibodies Scl-70 (indicative of diffuse systemic sclerosis), centromere (indicative of limited scleroderma), or Jo-1 (suggestive of poly/dermatomyositis).

4.9 A: All of the options

All of the options are associated with aggressive disease in rheumatoid arthritis. Other features include an elevated ESR, bony erosions on plain radiographs, and multiple joint involvement.

4.10 E: Start the patient on 60 mg/day oral prednisolone

Temporal arteritis, often associated with polymyalgia rheumatica, tends to occur abruptly and is commonly associated with either a temporal or occipital headache, scalp tenderness, constitutional symptoms, jaw claudication, and visual disturbance. In the presence of the latter, high-dose oral prednisolone should be commenced immediately to try and prevent visual loss from ischaemic optic neuropathy. A high ESR and histological evidence of arteritis are useful diagnostic tests. Although a biopsy is best performed as early as possible, the introduction of prednisolone should never be delayed.

The dose of steroid can be tapered downward slowly in steps of 5–10 mg every 2–4 weeks according to symptom control and a falling ESR. When the daily dose has reached 10 mg/day it is advised that a slower tapering regime be employed at 1 mg reductions every two weeks. Most patients will require daily maintenance doses of approximately 5 mg for 12 to 24 months. Some cases require longer term and higher dose maintenance therapy. In cases where this seems likely (prednisolone dose $\geq$ 7.5 mg/day for three months) prophylaxis against corticosteroid-induced osteoporosis should be started.

4.11   D: Measure spirochete antibodies

Lyme disease (LD) is a spirochaete (*B. burgdorferi*) tick-borne infection common throughout the world and in particular northern USA. The hallmark of LD is an annular erythamatous and often large (> 20 cm) rash (erythema chronicum migrans (ECM)) at the site of the tick bite. However, many people do not recall the bite or the rash. Constitutional symptoms of fever and fatigue may precede headaches, myalgia, arthralgia, tendonopathy, conjunctivitis, uveitis, pharyngitis, lymphadenopathy and testicular swelling.

Weeks later there may be cardiac or neurological symptoms and months later there may be a persistent inflammatory arthropathy and an atrophic rash of acrodermatitis chronica atrophicans.

Raised IgG or specific IgM antibodies to the spirochaete can be found 2–4 weeks after infection. The diagnosis is clinical, supported by this serological test.

Early disease is best treated with amoxycillin, doxycycline, or clarithromycin. Later cardiac, neurological, or persistent arthritic symptoms may also require a cephalosporin.

4.12   E: Warfarin should be dosed to maintain the INR at 2.0

Antiphospholipid syndrome is associated with recurrent venous and arterial thrombosis, spontaneous abortion, vasculitis, CNS disorders, and a 'catastrophic' widespread organ failure. Thrombocytopenia is seen in up to 25% of cases.

Antibodies are found in 5% of the general population and in association with several autoimmune rheumatic diseases (especially SLE), vasculitides, infection, and malignancy. Both the lupus anticoagulant and anticardiolipin antibodies should be measured though one and not the other may be present in up to 40% of cases. The lupus anticoagulant cannot be measured if the patient is already on heparin or warfarin.

Recurrent thrombosis should be treated with high-dose warfarin at an INR of 3–4.

4.13   C: Hypothyroidism

The following are recognised causes of ectopic calcification:

Hyperparathyroidism, hyperphosphataemia, sarcoidosis, hypervitaminosis D, tumour lysis, dermatomyositis, scleroderma

Ossification of soft-tissues occurs most often following traumatic myositis.

4.14   A: Churg Strauss syndrome

Other rheumatic diseases associated with pyoderma gangrenosum include systemic lupus erythematosus, Wegener's granulomatosis and sarcoidosis. Diabetes, haematological diseases such as leukaemia and myelofibrosis, and gastro-intestinal disorders including inflammatory bowel disease, chronic active hepatitis and primary biliary cirrhosis are also associated with the condition.

4.15   E: Raised parathyroid hormone

Pseudohypoparathyroidism (PHP) occurs as a result of target tissue resistance to parathyroid hormone (PTH). The biochemical consequences are hypocalcaemia, hyperphosphataemia and a raised PTH.

Pseudohypoparathyroidism may be tested for by measuring urine excretion of cyclic AMP (cAMP) in response to PTH. Administration of PTH to normal individuals leads to increased urinary excretion of cAMP. An abnormal response to this test in individuals with PHP classifies them either type I (no increase in urine cAMP) or type II (normal increase in urine cAMP but abnormal renal phosphate handling).

The clinical features of PHT include short stature, round facies, obesity, and brachydactyly. Pseudopseudohypoparathyroidism describes the clinical features in the presence of a normal serum calcium and PTH/cAMP test.

RHEUMATOLOGY: MULTIPLE CHOICE
ANSWERS

4.16   B C D

Around 70% of all rheumatoid arthritis patients, and 100% of those with nodules, are sero-positive for IgM rheumatoid factor. Secreted by B cells, the IgM factor reacts with the Fc component of IgG. The Rose-Waaler test uses sheep red cells coated with rabbit IgG. IgM factor is not specific to rheumatoid arthritis and may be seen in other disease and chronic infection.

4.17   A D E

Joint disease is characteristically non-erosive. Raynaud's disease is a feature in 50% of cases. Livido reticularis can be found in several conditions including bronchial and pancreatic carcinoma and polyarteritis nodosa. Hypertension and renal disease should be treated vigorously.

4.18   B C E

HLA-B27 is not usually helpful or reliable prognostically. The spondyloarthropathies can occur at any age but do so most often in young adults; spinal symptoms are more common in men. Synovitis is indistinguishable from that of rheumatoid arthritis but has a better prognosis and if transient is non-erosive. Eye lesions include conjunctivitis in 30% of patients with a 'reactive' arthritis but the overall incidence of uveitis generally is 5%. The iliitis of ankylosing spondylitis tends to be bilateral and that of psoriasis and Reiter's disease can be unilateral.

4.19   A B C D E

There is a strong (90%) female predominance. It is relatively rare in rheumatoid arthritis, but is common in SLE and Sjögren's disease. In scleroderma, Raynaud's phenomenon and nail fold capillary abnormalities with a positive ANA is a finding in 90% of cases destined to develop full systemic sclerosis. Treatment options include calcium channel blockers, ACE-inhibitors, gamolenic acid, prostacyclin and sympathectomy.

4.20   A B D E

Behçet's disease is twice as common in males. The mean age of onset is 30 years. The other important clinical feature is oro-genital ulceration. Venous thrombosis occurs in around 25% of cases. It is associated with HLA B5. Steroids and cyclosporin A are used in treatment.

4.21   A D

Aspiration of a suspected septic joint should be followed immediately by antibiotics pending a Gram stain and culture. A high white cell count and turbidity is non-specific; a high lactate suggests infection. *Staphylococcus aureus* accounts for 50% of infection; beta haemolytic *Streptococcus* 10%. The skin lesions of Lyme disease are best treated with tetracycline but the septic arthritis requires intravenous penicillin. About 20% of women with rubella can have a self-limiting, 'rheumatoid' like polyarthropathy which subsides after 6–8 weeks.

4.22   B D E

Steroid eye drops are not required and may be dangerous by predisposing to infection (particularly as a dry eye is prone to bacterial and fungal infection), scleral softening and perforation. The eye should be kept moist by regular use of artificial tears. Patients with some tear flow may benefit from electrocoagulation of the nasolacrimal glands to encourage the accumulation of residual tear drops. Other exocrine secretions, including those of the vagina, are affected, and the salivary glands may be enlarged typically in unilateral and episodic fashion. Most patients have the Anti-SS-A antibody named after the 'A' antigen of Sjögren's syndrome, now called anti-Ro.

4.23   D

Acute gout is treated with NSAIDs or colchicine. Aspirin, allopurinol and probenecid should be avoided initially. Blood urate corresponds poorly with clinical symptoms of gout and can be normal during an attack and raised in the asymptomatic; in this respect, hyperuricaemia *per se* is not an indication for allopurinol. Increased urate production is found in myeloproliferative disorders, high purine intake, obesity and excess alcohol and fructose consumption. A reduction in excretion is seen in intrinsic renal disease, with excess of metabolites (ketones, lactate) and with the use of thiazide diuretics. The causes of chondrocalcinosis include hypothyroidism, hypomagnesaemia, hypophosphatasia and haemochromatosis.

4.24   A D

Muscle weakness and tenderness are quite common and may contribute to the characteristic waddling gait. The bone volume is normal but undercalcified. The more potent forms of vitamin D are not required since uncomplicated osteomalacia is due to dietary deficiency and is therefore not resistant to treatment. The potent forms can be dangerous resulting in hypercalcaemia. Prolonged hypocalcaemia results in secondary hyperparathyroidism which can occasionally become autonomous. The bone scan is a useful way of detecting lesions since the decalcified bones avidly take up bone-seeking isotopes.

4.25   B E

The initial pathology in Paget's disease is abnormal resorption. Osteoclasts, via cytokines, stimulate osteoblastic remineralisation but the new bone architecture is not normal. Alkaline phosphatase (ALP) and hydroxyproline are good markers of bone turnover but ALP is not always raised in symptomatic patients. It is very rare to find new bone involvement after the initial diagnosis other than some spread along those bones already affected. The bisphosphonates are analogues of pyrophosphate and inhibit osteoclastic activity. Etidronate in high doses can inhibit osteoblasts and induce osteomalacia.

4.26   C

The triad of urethritis, conjunctivitis and arthritis is characteristic; added to this is buccal ulceration and balanitis and 20% have sacro-iliitis. About 1% of patients with a non-specific urethritis develop Reiter's syndrome. The disease is often not self-limiting and may progress with 80% of patients having symptoms at 5 years.

4.27   A B D E

Privational causes include food fads and poor diet intake of vitamin D. Gastrointestinal disturbances including gastrectomy, malabsorption and liver disease can all lead to osteomalacia. The renal tubular diseases have high phosphate clearance in common and chronic renal failure (not acute) leads to a decreased production of 1,25 dihydroxy vitamin D.

4.28   C D

Osteogenesis imperfecta (OI) occurs in 1 in 30,000 births. It is a disorder of bone type I collagen and all except type III OI are autosomal dominant. Type I and IV OI are the more common variants and relatively benign; type IV have normal sclerae. Type III OI is associated with progressive severe disease and multiple fractures. Type II is non-viable. Other features include abnormal dentine and ossicles, hypermobility, tendon rupture and leaky heart valves.

4.29   A B C D E

Several endocrinopathies can cause osteoporosis; others to consider are thyrotoxicosis, hyperparathyroidism and hypogonadism. Other drugs associated with the condition are steroids, heparin and cytotoxics. Conditions such as myeloma lead to osteoporosis partly by a local infiltrative affect but also by cytokine stimulation of bone resorption.

4.30   A B E

The typical features of PMR outside the musculoskeletal system are depression and weight loss. There may also be low-grade fever. If temporal arteritis supervenes there may also be headache and facial pain. The presence of lymphadenopathy should alert one to the possibility of a paraneoplastic syndrome, which may present with similar clinical features. Muscle enzymes are raised in polymyositis which is associated with muscle fibril destruction. It is increasingly recognised that there may be synovitis in patients with PMR particularly affecting the shoulders and sternoclavicular joints. Occasionally there may also be peripheral synovitis in the small joints of the hands resembling rheumatoid arthritis.

CLINICAL PHARMACOLOGY: REVISION CHECKLIST

Interactions/dose adjustment

- ☐ Drug interactions
- ☐ Pregnancy/breast feeding
- ☐ Adverse effects – general
- ☐ Dose adjustment in renal failure
- ☐ Drugs in porphyria
- ☐ Polymorphism of drug metabolism

Specific side-effects of drugs

- ☐ Asthma exacerbation
- ☐ Causing hypothyroidism
- ☐ Gynaecomastia/ hyperprolactinaemia
- ☐ Hepatic enzyme inducers
- ☐ Hypokalaemia
- ☐ Aggravation of skin disorders
- ☐ Convulsions
- ☐ Haemolytic anaemia

Fundamental pharmacology

- ☐ Mechanisms of drug/antibiotic action

Most frequently considered individual agents

- ☐ Antipsychotics/depressants
- ☐ ACE inhibitors
- ☐ Amiodarone
- ☐ Thiazides
- ☐ Anti-convulsants
- ☐ Digoxin
- ☐ Lithium
- ☐ Sulfasalazine
- ☐ Metronidazole
- ☐ Radio-iodine

Other 'topical' agents

- ☐ Azidothymidine (AZT)
- ☐ Cimetidine
- ☐ Gentamicin
- ☐ Griseofulvin
- ☐ HMG Co-A reductase inhibitor
- ☐ L-dopa
- ☐ Metronidazole
- ☐ Penicillamine
- ☐ Retinoic acid
- ☐ Warfarin

IMMUNOLOGY: REVISION CHECKLIST

Cytokines

☐ Tumour necrosis factor

☐ Interferon

☐ Inflammatory mediators (general)

☐ Leukotrienes

Cellular immunity

☐ T lymphocytes/deficiency

☐ Cell-mediated immunity

Immunoglobulins/autoimmunity

☐ IgA/IgE/IgG

☐ Autoimmune disease/ANCA

☐ Hypogammaglobulinaemia

☐ Monoclonal gammopathy

☐ Tissue receptor antibodies

☐ Circulating immune complexes

☐ Precipitating antibodies in diagnosis

Miscellaneous

☐ Complement/CH_{50}

☐ Angioneurotic oedema

☐ Hypersensitivity reactions

☐ Mast cells

☐ Polymerase chain reaction

☐ Post-splenectomy

☐ Transplant rejection

INFECTIOUS DISEASES: REVISION CHECKLIST

Viral Infections

☐ Hepatitis

☐ Infectious mononucleosis

☐ Chickenpox/measles/mumps

☐ AIDS/HIV

☐ Adenovirus

☐ Genital herpes

☐ Parvovirus

Bacterial Infections

☐ Venereal disease

☐ Brucellosis

☐ TB/BCG

☐ Tetanus

☐ Toxoplasmosis

☐ Typhoid/cholera

☐ Bacteroides

☐ *Haemophilus influenza*

☐ *Helicobacter pylori*

☐ Lyme disease

☐ Meningitis

☐ Pneumonia

☐ Staphylococcus

Routes of infection

☐ Transmission by insect bite

☐ Faecal-oral transmission

Tropical and protozoal infections

- ☐ Malaria
- ☐ Tropical fever/splenomegaly
- ☐ Giardiasis
- ☐ *Pneumocystis carinii*
- ☐ Schistosomiasis

Miscellaneous

- ☐ *Chlamydia trachomatis*
- ☐ Other infections/diarrhoea
- ☐ Chronic infection and anaemia
- ☐ Infections and eosinophilia
- ☐ Prion disease

RHEUMATOLOGY: REVISION CHECKLIST

Auto-immune disease

- [ ] Rheumatoid arthritis
- [ ] SLE
- [ ] Wegener's granulomatosis

Other vasculitides

- [ ] Polymyalgia rheumatica
- [ ] Cranial arteritis
- [ ] Vasculitic disease

Other arthritides

- [ ] Reiter's syndrome
- [ ] Ankylosing spondylitis/HLA B27
- [ ] Arthralgia
- [ ] Behçet's disease
- [ ] Arthropathy (general)
- [ ] Hypertrophic osteo-arthropathy
- [ ] Osteoarthritis
- [ ] Pseudogout

Miscellaneous

- [ ] Anti-phospholipid syndrome
- [ ] Digital gangrene
- [ ] Peri-articular calcification
- [ ] Systemic sclerosis

INDEX

Numbers refer to question numbers.

Clinical Pharmacology

Immunology

Infectious Diseases

Rheumatology

PASTEST BOOKS FOR MRCP PART 1

MRCP 1 New Pocket Series
Further titles in this range:
Book 1:   Cardiology, Haematology, Respiratory   *1901198 758*
Book 2:   Basic Sciences, Neurology, Psychiatry   *1901198 804*
Book 3:   Endocrinology, Gastroenterology, Nephrology   *1901198 855*

MRCP 1 New 'Best of Five' Multiple Choice Revision Book
K Binymin   *1901198 57X*
Our new 'Best of Five' Multiple Choice Revision book features subject-based chapters ensuring all topics are fully covered. Practise new format 'best of five' questions to give confidence in your ability to sit the exam.

MRCP 1 Multiple True/False Revision Book
P Kalra   *1901198 952*
This book brings together 600 PasTest multiple true/false questions into one volume. The book is split into subjects but also contains a practice exam so that you can test your knowledge. Again, detailed teaching notes are provided.

Essential Revision Notes for MRCP Revised Edition
P Kalra   *1901198 596*
A definitive guide to revision for the MRCP examination. 19 chapters of informative material necessary to gain a successful exam result.

Explanations to the RCP 1997 and 1998 Past Papers
G Rees   *1901198 286*
360 answers and teaching notes to the Royal College of Physicians book of MCQs from the MRCP Part 1 1997 and 1998 Examinations.

Explanations to the RCP 1990 Past Papers
H Beynon & C Ross   *1901198 576*
180 answers and teaching notes to the Royal College of Physicians book of MCQs from the MRCP Part 1 1990 Examinations.

MRCP Part 1 MCQs with Key Topic Summaries 2nd edition
P O'Neill   *1901198 073*
200 MCQs with comprehensive key topic summaries bridging the gap between standard MCQ books and textbooks.

MRCP Part 1 MCQs in Basic Sciences
P Easterbrook & K Mokbel   *1901198 347*
300 exam-based MCQs focusing on basic sciences, with answers and teaching notes.

PASTEST – DEDICATED TO YOUR SUCCESS

PasTest has been publishing books for doctors for over 25 years. Our extensive experience means that we are always one step ahead when it comes to knowledge of current trends and content of the Royal College exams.

We use only the best authors and lecturers, many of whom are Consultants and Royal College Examiners, which enables us to tailor our books and courses to meet your revision needs. We incorporate feedback from candidates to ensure that our books are continually improved.

This commitment to quality ensures that students who buy a PasTest book or attend a PasTest course achieve successful exam results.

100% Money Back Guarantee

We're sure you will find our study books invaluable, but in the unlikely event that you are not entirely happy, we will give you your money back – guaranteed.

Delivery to your Door

With a busy lifestyle, nobody enjoys walking to the shops for something that may or may not be in stock. Let us take the hassle and deliver direct to your door. We will despatch your book within 24 hours of receiving your order. We also offer free delivery on books for medical students to UK addresses.

How to Order:

 ## www.pastest.co.uk

To order books safely and securely online, shop online at our website.

☎ Telephone: +44 (0)1565 752000

Fill out the order form as a helpful prompt and have your credit card to hand when you call.

✉ PasTest Ltd, FREEPOST, Knutsford, WA16 7BR.

Send your completed order form with your cheque (made payable to PasTest Ltd) and debit or credit card details to the above address. (Please complete your address details on the reverse of the cheque.)

 +44 (0)1565 650264

Fax your completed order form with your debit or credit card details.

WMD 3 0 0 4 0 3